Praying for a Cure

Point/Couterpoint
Philosophers Debate Contemporary Issues
Series Editors: James P. Sterba and Rosemarie Tong

This new series provides a philosophical angle to debates currently raging in academic and larger circles. Each book is a short volume (around 200 pages) in which two or more prominent philosophers debate different sides of an issue. For more information contact Professor Sterba, Department of Philosophy, University of Notre Dame, Notre Dame IN 46566, or Professor Tong, Department of Philosophy, Davidson College, Davidson, NC 28036.

Praying for a Cure

When Medical and Religious Practices Conflict

Peggy DesAutels
Margaret P. Battin
Larry May

ROWMAN & LITTLEFIELD PUBLISHERS, INC.
Lanham • Boulder • New York • Oxford

ROWMAN & LITTLEFIELD PUBLISHERS, INC.

Published in the United States of America
by Rowman & Littlefield Publishers, Inc.
4720 Boston Way, Lanham, Maryland 20706

12 Hid's Copse Road
Cumnor Hill, Oxford OX2 9JJ, England

British Library Cataloguing in Publication Information Available

Library of Congress Cataloging-in-Publication Data

DesAutels, Peggy, 1955–
   Praying for a cure : when medical and religious practices conflict
/ Peggy DesAutels, Margaret P. Battin, Larry May
     p. cm.—(Point/counterpoint)
   Includes bibliographical references and index.
   ISBN 0-8476-9262-0 (alk. paper).—ISBN 0-8476-9263-9 (paper :
alk. paper)
   1. Christian Science—Doctrines. 2. Spiritual healing.
3. Health—Religious aspects—Christian Science. 4. Medicine—
Religious aspects—Christian Science. 5. Christian Science—
Controversial literature. I. Battin, M. Pabst. II. May, Larry.
III. Title. IV. Series.
BX6950.D47 1999
261.5'61'088285—dc21   98-45358
                                                      CIP

Printed in the United States of America

♾ ™The paper used in this publication meets the minimum requirements of
American National Standard for Information Sciences—Permanence of Paper for
Printed Library Materials, ANSI Z39.48–1984.

Contents

Acknowledgments

Peggy DesAutels is grateful to Margaret Walker for encouraging her to take on this project and offering many insights and ideas as the book took shape. Thanks go to Robert Richardson for his willingness to read and respond to numerous earlier drafts and to Joan Callahan, Peter French, Laurie Calhoun, Carl Becker, Karen Grayson, David Nartonis, Mary Lu Fennell, and Tom Fennell for their helpful comments.

The Ethics Center at the University of South Florida supported this project in a number of ways, providing a stimulating and supportive work environment. Kathy Agne's skilled, timely, and always cheerful support at the center was especially appreciated. Thanks also go to the Christian Science Committee on Publication, The First Church of Christ, Scientist, Boston, Massachusetts, for providing information on the activities and views of the Christian Science Church.

Peggy DesAutels appreciates the full support she receives from her family, especially Lane and Travis DesAutels, for her academic endeavors.

Peggy DesAutels, Peggy Battin, and Larry May would like to thank many colleagues with whom we have discussed these isues, both at the 1996 AMINTAPHIL meetings in Lexington, KY, and elsewhere–including Ken Kipnis, Joan Callahan, Richard DeGeorge, Hamner Hill, Mike W. Martin, and Phil Quinn. We would also like to thank the publishers who allowed us to print revised versions of the following essays:

"High-Risk Religion," by Margaret Pabst Battin, chapter 2 of *Ethics in the Sanctuary: Examining the Practices of Organized Religion* (New Haven: Yale University Press, 1990). By permission of the publisher.

"Christian Science, Rational Choice, and Alternative World Views," by Peggy DesAutels, *Journal of Social Philosophy* 26, no. 3 (Winter 1995). By permission of the publisher.

"Put Up or Shut Up? A Reply to Peggy DesAutels' Defense of Christian Science," by Margaret Battin, *Journal of Social Philosophy* 26, no. 3 (Winter 1995): By permission of the publisher.

"Challenging Medical Authority: The Refusal of Treatment by Christian Scientists," by Larry May, *Hastings Center Report,* January-February 1995, by permission of the publisher, and chapter 9 of *The Socially Responsive Self* (Chicago: University of Chicago Press, 1996). By permission of the publisher.

Introduction

Peggy DesAutels, Margaret P. Battin, and Larry May

Three recent and sometimes conflicting trends have contributed to renewed public concern and debate over health-related religious practices. First, more and more people are acknowledging and even insisting on a patient's right to make his or her own health- and death-related choices. Second, there has been an increasing (though reluctant) acknowledgment by the medical community of the effectiveness of alternative approaches to healing, including religious approaches, for at least some types of people with some types of diseases. And third, the state has become increasingly involved in "protecting" vulnerable populations such as children, the elderly, and the disabled.

Because of increased recognition of a patient's right to refuse conventional medical treatments and to seek alternative healing methods, it is now widely accepted by medical ethicists and the courts that competent adults may refuse life-saving treatments on religious grounds. But can parents refuse medical treatment for their children? Although neither a legal nor an ethical consensus has been reached on this question, there has been increased public concern over (as well as state interference in) a wide variety of types of cases of apparent child neglect and abuse. Whether medical refusals for children are tantamount to child abuse has not yet been legally determined. In fact, in various cases across the country in which children have died as a result of their parents' exclusive reliance on a religious cure, the charges against such parents have ranged from no charges at all to neglect to child endangerment to manslaughter to murder.

This volume focuses the debate over the ethics surrounding conflicting religious and medical practices by examining the specific case of health-related choices made by and for Christian Scientists. Although there are several religious groups who refuse medical treatment or components of it, the issues surrounding Christian Scientists' medical refusals are especially vexing and ethically complex. Many of us are vaguely familiar with the fact that "Christian Scientists are the ones who do not go to doctors," but few know much more about how a Christian Scientist's view of the world conflicts with that of the majority; nor do many of us know much about the substantive ethical issues surrounding a Christian Scientist's health-related choices.

There are several reasons for delving more deeply into the political, social, and ethical conflicts that arise from the practice of Christian Science. First, medical professionals in clinical settings are likely to encounter a variety of diverging cultures and worldviews that incorporate approaches to health and healing that clash with medical approaches. The culture and worldview of Christian Scientists is a good case in point. Second, our society must decide how tolerant it should be toward minority groups, religious or otherwise, with defining practices that challenge the moral convictions of the majority. Christian Science children's cases do tend, at least prima facie, to challenge one of our deepest moral convictions that children should not be allowed to suffer or die. And third, because Christian Scientists tend to be well-educated professionals who generally make rational, well-informed choices in their lives, their health-related choices cannot simply be dismissed as choices made by irrational fanatics. Rather, a determination of the rationality of their choices can only be made after an in-depth critical examination of their views and practices.

This volume addresses the issues surrounding the health-related choices of Christian Scientists in a rather unique way. It has a point-counterpoint format but contains three voices rather than the usual two. The three authors of this book are philosophers who work in overlapping areas of philosophy but take very different stands. Peggy DesAutels has published in the areas of medical ethics, moral psychology, and philosophy of mind. Peggy Battin has published in bioethics, aesthetics, health policy, professional ethics, and in particular on end-of-life issues. Larry May has published in philosophy of law, theory of moral responsibility, and professional ethics. Battin and May are not Christian Scientists; DesAutels was raised in this tradition.

High-Risk Religions and Informed Consent

In the first half of the book, Peggy DesAutels and Margaret P. Battin examine certain religious practices by drawing on concepts and norms from professional ethics, rational choice theory, and philosophy of science. The religious practices of concern to them involve the ways in which some religious institutions influence their members to make "high-risk" decisions.

More specifically, they address the following questions: Why do members of the Christian Science church uniformly take health-related risks that other people do not? And is the Christian Science church ethically irresponsible in the ways it influences its members' decision-making processes?

DesAutels and Battin differ over whether the Christian Science Church is ethically remiss for failing to supply healing success-rate statistics to its adherents. Battin claims that the Christian Science Church is morally culpable for publishing only anecdotal accounts of healing successes because its members are then unable to assess the risks involved in choosing a Christian Science approach to healing. She argues that the Christian Science Church systematically disregards the principle of autonomy and violates requirements of informed consent by providing to its adherents only selected accounts of successful cures. DesAutels, on the other hand, defends the practice of publishing only healing successes. She argues that the Christian Scientist's decision to pursue spiritual means for treatment does not resemble in structure the decision to pursue a particular medical treatment and that therefore cure-rate information is inapplicable to a Christian Scientist's decision-making process.

Christian Science in a Pluralistic Society

In the second half of the book, Peggy DesAutels and Larry May debate how to treat the seemingly harmful practices of a minority religion within a larger pluralistic, secular society. May considers the stalemate that can arise between Christian Scientists and medical professionals over the treatment of Christian Science children to be primarily a conflict of groups over authority within a pluralistic society. He takes a communitarian perspective on the question: In a pluralistic society such as ours, at what point should respect for a religious minority culture be tempered by concerns for the fundamental rights of children? May argues that neither the medical community nor the Christian Science community should be given exclusive purview in determining the best means for securing a child's right to health. Rather, the two groups should compromise. Christian Scientists should be socialized to be more open to medical diagnoses in order better to know when to seek medical help for their children in life-threatening situations, and medical professionals should be socialized to be more sensitive to patients as persons and more open to nonstandard approaches to health in non-life-threatening situations.

DesAutels responds by claiming that the conflicts that arise between Christian Scientists and medical professionals are best described not as a conflict over authority but as a conflict over worldviews. She maintains that the fundamental disagreement between members of the two groups rests on the significant disparities between a religious idealist belief system and a secular materialist belief system. No compromise is possible between two such different worldviews. Because neither group intends that children suffer and both groups value the health of children, the two groups should simply respect each other's disparate worldviews and resulting health-related choices.

Practices, Beliefs, and Church Structure of Christian Scientists

Christian Scientists rarely, if ever, go to doctors. They usually choose instead to rely exclusively on prayer for healing. One major difference between a Christian Scientist's approach to praying for healing and that taken by more mainstream Christian denominations is that Christian Scientists do not attempt to "mix" prayer with a medical approach. They view the two approaches—prayer versus medicine—as incompatible. Christian Science doctrine does not *forbid* going to doctors. Rather, it is up to each Christian Scientist to decide whether to use a Christian Science prayer-based approach or a medical approach.

Because Christian Scientists choose to take such a radical stand on health-related issues and because they commit to a lifestyle so different from most, their choice to be Christian Scientists is usually a carefully considered one. They do not deem themselves to be Christian Scientists simply by virtue of their choice of church on Sunday. Even those whose upbringing included faithful attendance at a Christian Science church must eventually choose for themselves whether to make the significant commitment to a way of life that includes, among other things, daily prayer and study, no drinking, and no smoking.

The Christian Science view of prayer is different from that of some "faith-healing" religions. For Christian Scientists, it is an ongoing process of better understanding and demonstrating that there is a perfect spiritual order already in existence. They believe that when this order is felt and understood, suffering in human experience is overcome and eliminated. Thus prayer is not viewed as a petition to God to intervene by performing a miracle of some sort. Rather, prayer is a search for an increased understanding of spiritual reality—a search that, when successful, results in the exemplification of this reality in one's experience. When praying about a specific situation, Christian Scientists mentally affirm relevant spiritual facts and deny the ultimate reality of anything that appears to contradict these facts.

In philosophical terms, Christian Scientists are idealists. Mary Baker Eddy, the woman who founded Christian Science in the 1860s, reasoned that if God, infinite Mind, is All, then there is no matter. What is perceived by humans as a physical universe is, in reality, nothing more than the conscious and unconscious thoughts of mortals. As Richard Nenneman, a Christian Scientist and past editor of the *Christian Science Monitor*, explains it, the physical universe is "ultimately unreal, but it is, in terms of the human perception of it, also plastic—it is molded according to the thinking brought to bear on it by each individual."[1] In other words, for Christian Scientists, the experience of inharmonious physical conditions (e.g., disease) is illusory and temporary. Their view is that a better understanding of God's harmonious spiritual universe will cause an apparently unhealthy physical condition to change into a healthy, harmonious "physical" condition. Prayer, then, is not just an optimistic hope "in the patient's mind" but is, for Christian Scientists, a better grasp of the loving and good nature of ultimate reality. This better understanding is exemplified on the patient's body, since for a Christian Scientist, the patient's body is itself nothing more than an image in thought.

Christian Scientists refer to themselves as "Christian" because they study and attempt to follow the teachings and example of Jesus. But their conception of Jesus' relation to God differs from that of most other Christian denominations. The human Jesus is, for Christian Scientists, an exemplar and way show-er, but Jesus' relationship to God is seen as being no different from any other human's. Jesus merely expressed and demonstrated God's ever-presence more fully than any other human being has before or since. Thus, Christian Scientists think that anyone can heal just as Jesus did by emulating his way of life and better understanding his teachings.

The structure of the Christian Science Church also differs from that of many mainstream Christian denominations. There are no Christian Science ministers or clergy. Instead, church services are conducted by two "readers" who are elected from within each church's congregation to serve for two or three years. Sunday services incorporate readings from the Bible and the Christian Science "textbook," *Science and Health with Key to the Scriptures,* by Mary Baker Eddy.[2] Wednesday evening services also include time for members of the congregation to share recent healing experiences or thoughts on Christian Science. Rules for governing both the central or "Mother" church, in Boston, Massachusetts, and its branch churches throughout the United States and the world, are found in the *Church Manual.*[3]

When Christian Scientists desire assistance or guidance from other Christian Scientists, they have several options. If they would like someone to pray for them, they can call on a Christian Science "practitioner." Practitioners charge for their services and are listed in the *Christian Science Journal,* a monthly publication. They are well versed in the teachings of Christian Science and are required to submit evidence of healing effectiveness to the Mother Church prior to being listed. If Christian Scientists wish to learn more about how to practice the teachings of Christian Science in their day-to-day lives, they can apply for what is termed "class instruction." These two-week classes are taught by "teachers" of Christian Science. Practitioners who have been especially successful at prayer-based healing and have gone through an additional course from a current teacher of Christian Science are eligible themselves to become teachers. Trained Christian Science nurses are also available for those who need nursing services. Unlike practitioners and teachers, nurses do not pray for their patients and, unlike medical nurses, they do not administer any sort of medication. Instead, they assist with daily hygiene, dress wounds, and keep patients as comfortable as possible while the patient addresses the situation through prayer. Most major cities in the United States have several Christian Science churches (First Church of Christ, Scientist; Second Church of Christ Scientist; and so on). Many also have a Christian Science nursing facility.

As specific issues and controversies arise in the course of this volume's debate, additional details on Christian Science views and practices are brought to bear. However, the authors of this volume do not pretend to offer a complete exposition of either Christian Science theology or the Christian Science way of life. Instead, they hope to expand a new field within applied philosophy—one in which the ethics surrounding the views, values, and practices found within an organized religion are reflectively and critically examined by both those within the religion and those who stand outside it.

Notes

1. Richard A. Nenneman, *The New Birth of Christianity: Why Religion Persists in a Scientific Age* (San Francisco: HarperCollins, 1992), 155–156.

2. Mary Baker Eddy, *Science and Health with Key to the Scriptures* (1875; Boston: The First Church of Christ, Scientist, 1934).

3. Mary Baker Eddy, *Manual of The Mother Church, The First Church of Christ, Scientist in Boston, Massachusetts,* 89th ed. (Boston: The First Church of Christ, Scientist, 1895).

1

High-Risk Religion: Christian Science and the Violation of Informed Consent

Margaret P. Battin

In some of the more colorful groups on the American religious spectrum, the religious faith of believers involves a willingness to take substantial physical risks—risks to health and physical functioning, even the risk of death. In several of these groups, the risks a believer takes are indirect, as in refusing blood transfusions or other medical treatment; in others, the risks are direct and immediate, as in drinking strychnine or handling poisonous snakes. Christian Science, as the Church of Christ, Scientist, is informally called, is one of these groups: Its members refuse virtually all medical treatment for illness or disease, relying instead on Christian Science's distinctive practice of "healing."

We may think of these practices as extraordinary tests of religious commitment. A willingness to risk death seems to exhibit the extraordinary value religion can have for believers; indeed, willingness to risk death for religious reasons is often extolled as the highest test of faith. But this willingness also raises a set of disturbing moral issues concerning the ways in which religious groups encourage their adherents to take such risks.

In what follows, I want to take a closer look at the influence of religious groups on their adherents' choices, focusing on high-risk decision making that can result in death, particularly in Christian Science. The same sorts of issues arise for many other groups as well: Jehovah's Witnesses; the Indiana-based Faith Assembly; the serpent-handling, strychnine-drinking Holiness churches of the Appalachian Mountains; the Oklahoma-Colorado Church of the First Born; End Time Ministries in South

Dakota; the Pennsylvania-based Faith Tabernacle; the Oregon City, Oregon, group the Followers of Christ; and others.[1] I do not wish to suggest that the willingness of believers in these groups to risk death may not be sincere and devout; rather, I want to cast a morally inquiring eye on the way in which religious institutions engender these sincere, devout beliefs. Christian Science, I shall argue, is among the most problematic of these.

This characterization may seem to be at odds with the social position of Christian Science. It is sometimes claimed in defense of Christian Science that its members tend to be upper-income, well-educated, professional people who are stable members of society, nonusers of drugs, alcohol, or tobacco—solid citizens, reliable and trustworthy. This is not a group on the margins of society or one scrabbled together by taking advantage of unfortunates with serious social or psychological problems. Yet, I shall argue, the practices of the Christian Science church nevertheless constitute a continuing violation of one of the most basic ordinary and professional moral norms, the requirement of *informed consent* when individuals are asked or invited to take risks to their own health or lives.

Risk Budgets and Styles

How do people come to take risks? How may other persons and institutions influence someone to take risks he or she might otherwise not accept? Is there something distinctive (or troubling) about a religious group that encourages its members to take risks—risks with their health, risks with their lives? To pose the problem in a precise way, we can conceptualize the issue of high-risk religion as it might be addressed in the field of professional ethics. Drawing on issues concerning the formation and manipulation of choice, especially in medicine, we can approach this problem under the general rubric of *informed consent,* thus applying norms from professional ethics to practices within organized religion.

In everyday life, risks that a person voluntarily and knowingly takes can be described as the result of a prudential calculation, however rudimentary that calculation may be in practice, in which he or she elects a course of action hoping it will produce a gain or avoid a loss while recognizing that it may either concurrently or alternatively result in a (further) loss. This prudential calculation involves a survey of the range of possible outcomes of the action proposed, an assessment of the likelihood of the various possible outcomes (the decision is made *under risk* if the probabilities are known, *under uncertainty* if they are not), and an assessment of the relative desirability or undesirability of each of the possible outcomes. Typically, avoidance risk taking weighs two or more projected negative outcomes against each other; gain-oriented, positive risk taking may weigh various positive outcomes against each other, or a positive outcome against both the cost of failing to achieve it and the cost of failing to take the risk. Whatever the specific context of the risk decision, the decision maker properly makes the calculation by multiplying the value of each possible outcome times the probability that it will occur, if known (or the best approximation to it), and then choosing the course of action promising the highest expected utility. That this calculation may be made in a completely intuitive, nonquantitative way does not obscure its nature: Conscious decision making under risk or under uncertainty always involves acting so as to produce some preferred outcome while recognizing that this action may instead produce a different, undesired result.

Each individual, Charles Fried has pointed out, has a distinctive *risk budget*—the degree and severity of risk he or she is willing to accept in order to avoid certain losses or to achieve certain gains.[2] The risk budget is a function of the possible courses of action the individual foresees, the probabilities he or she assigns to the various possible outcomes, and the utilities he or she attaches to each of these, influenced by any characteristic errors the person may make in performing the prudential calculation that indicates what course of action promises the greatest expected utility. Although the risk budgets of ordinary individuals in a culture appear to be fairly uniform with respect to the background risks of everyday life (e.g., in drinking the water in a given locality or in using electricity in one's home), there is considerable divergence in the willingness of individuals to accept specific higher foreground risks—for instance, in financial dealings or in high-risk sports like hang gliding or mountain climbing. This is just to say that some members of a culture take risks that other members of the culture won't.

Furthermore, each individual has a distinctive *risk style*—the degree of deliberation or abandon he or she exercises in making a prudential calculation under risk or uncertainty. Some people assess perceived risks with meticulous, painstaking care, regardless of whether the risks are mild or severe and the amount of information they have about the probabilities of various possible outcomes; other take both big and little risks in a comparatively cavalier way. Different individuals also process relevant information in very different ways. For instance, some are naturally optimistic, focusing primarily on the benefits to be gained; other are comparatively pessimistic, attending to possible losses, even when their estimates of the probabilities of the outcomes are the same. In processing information, some individuals may be more prone to characteristic errors of reasoning in risk assessment than others. Like risk budgets, the risk styles of persons within a culture are relatively uniform with respect to background risks but may vary considerably among individuals with respect to certain more conspicuous risks. Some people make their choices about risks in ways that other people would regard as foolish.

The problem presented by the practices of Christian Science, as well as other high-risk religious groups, arises with an observation about risk budgets and styles. The members of a culture ordinarily exhibit broad commonalities in both risk budgets and styles with respect to background risks; they also typically exhibit a range of idiosyncratic, individual risk budgets and styles with respect to certain conspicuous, higher-risk decisions. However, the risk budgets and styles of the members of certain religious groups display striking uniformities not so much with respect to background risks but with respect to major, conspicuous foreground risks—direct risks to health, physical functions, and even risks to life. Furthermore, the kinds of risk characteristically taken by members of these groups often fall well outside the risk budgets and, in addition, violate the risk styles of most other members of society, even outside the quite broad range of individual variation in risk budget and style that members of the culture ordinarily display in their decisions. Put another way, the members of certain religious groups like Christian Science take risks other people do not and decide to do so in ways that other people would not, but they nevertheless do so in remarkably uniform ways. Nor are these trivial risks; some are potentially fatal ones.

These characteristic risk-taking patterns, each distinctive of a particular group, may seem to be just another element in the colorful spectrum of American religious diversity. But this diversity cloaks substantial moral issues about the ways in which religious groups influence and shape individual decision making among their members. It is not merely that these people take risks other people do not and decide to do so in ways other people would not; it is the very uniformity of these group-specific risk budgets and styles and the degree to which they fall outside the ordinary range of variation that invites scrutiny of the mechanisms by which they are produced. What we will find in these religious groups—including Christian Science—are systematic, doctrine-controlled violations of the principle of autonomy, that is, of the moral principle familiar in professional and ordinary ethics that requires both protection of an individual's capacity to choose and respect for the substance of that choice.

If there are violations of the principle of autonomy, they can be identified by locating the precise point at which they occur in the paradigmatic decision-making process, evident in varying forms in different religious groups whose adherents regularly make choices that indirectly or directly expose them to risks of death. Are these choices *informed?* Do they involve *consent,* genuine consent that is voluntary and uncoerced? In answering these questions (questions that can be articulated more clearly in part because we are approaching the problem from the standpoint of professional ethics), we will come to see that at least some of the ways in which religious groups shape and control high-risk decision making are morally indefensible.

Risk Taking in Christian Science

The First Church of Christ, Scientist, takes the refusal of conventional medical treatment in favor of Christian Science healing as central among its practices and as indicative of faith.[3] According to Christian Science belief, what we (mistakenly) call "disease" is produced by a "radically limited and distorted view of the true spiritual nature and capacities of men and women."[4] "Illness" results from "human alienation from God,"[5] produced by fundamental misunderstanding. Disease is symptomatic not of physical disorder but of underlying spiritual inadequacy and a failure to understand one's true spiritual nature. A faithful member of the church who falls ill consults a Christian Science practitioner to seek treatment, which consists "entirely of heartfelt yet disciplined prayer."[6] The practitioner, who is often consulted by telephone (sometimes long distance) and need not make a bedside visit, has no medical training in either diagnosis or treatment. The practitioner does not physically touch or examine the patient. Rather, the practitioner assists the ill person in prayer, the objective of which is to relieve physical symptoms by promoting the correct and reverent understanding of the true nature of disease: In reality there is no such thing. Prayer is believed to be incompatible with conventional medical treatment, since a medical treatment presupposes the misleading assumption that there is such a thing as disease, that it is of physical origin, and that it can be treated by physical means. Properly, one cannot speak of *cure,* for there is no disease to be cured; rather, the relief of symptoms is a "demonstration" of the correctness of the principles upon which Christian Science is founded. Christian Scientists do generally use the services of dentists and oculists and sometimes have physicians perform what they call "mechanical" procedures not involving medication, such as setting broken bones; but other than this, no conventional medical procedures, either diagnostic or therapeutic, are used.[7] For services rendered in praying for and with the individual who is ill, the Christian Science practitioner receives a fee roughly comparable to the fees conventional physicians charge. This fee is reimbursable by many insurance companies (including some Blue Cross/Blue Shield plans) and by some state and federal Medicare and Medicaid programs.[8] There are about 2,800 Christian Science practitioners who practice healing through prayer on a full-time basis and about 675 nurses listed in the *Christian Science Journal.*[9]

Frequently, the choice between Christian Science healing and conventional medical treatment does not constitute a subjectively recognized *risk* for the devout Scientist, since belief in the efficacy of Christian Science healing may be very strong. In such cases, the individual may be confident that Christian Science healing will provide relief from the condition that troubles him. Nevertheless, the choice to accept treatment from a Christian Science practitioner rather than a medical doctor, or not to accept treatment at all, resembles in structure any other prudential calculation under risk: Various possible outcomes—cure, continuing illness, incapacitation, and death—are foreseen under specific valuations and under more or less quantifiable expectations about the likelihood of their occurrence. Christian Scientists are, of course, aware of the availability of conventional medicine; medical treatment is a possible choice, but one that, on prudential grounds, the believing Christian Scientist does not make. The believing Scientist not only thinks he or she is acting in accord with the dictates or expectations of the faith but also that he or she will maximize the likelihood of achieving the outcome with the greatest expected utility, namely, a successful cure, by preferring Christian Science healing to conventional medicine. It is in this choice that the risk taking lies; the believing Christian Scientist, of course, sees it as a good risk.

Christian Science is not the only religious group whose high-risk practices challenge the principle of informed consent. Others include Jehovah's Witnesses, who refuse a single component of medical treatment—the transfusion of blood or blood derivatives into their bodies—on the basis of scriptural passages that prohibit eating or drinking blood; the Faith Assembly, a small fundamentalist group centered in northwestern Indiana, which at its height prohibited members from consulting doctors or using any medical treatment at all, including vaccination, assistance in childbirth, emergency treatment, prostheses, eyeglasses, or hearing aids; and the Holiness churches, widespread in the Appalachian regions of the southeastern United States, many of which practice serpent handling and strychnine drinking on the basis of biblical directives, and others named at the outset: the Church of the First Born, End Time Ministries, the Faith Tabernacle, and the Followers of Christ, all of which teach avoidance of medical care. But Christian Science is the one I want to focus on here, in part because its practices are particularly problematic.

Altering Risk Budgets

Even when the risk taker's prudential calculation is neither skewed by the imposition of coercively large costs for failing to take the risk nor made in an emotionally heightened condition, there are two further ways this calculation can be distorted. Like any other group, a religious group can influence the individual's estimate of the probability of the various outcomes he or she foresees, or it can change the evaluations assigned by the individual to these outcomes, or both. In both cases, the effect of the influence is not to coerce choice or to impair its quality by altering risk style but to alter the individual's risk budget.

Altering Assessments of Probabilities

A person reasonably conversant with the circumstances of the world knows certain facts: that malnourishment impairs health, that rattlesnakes are poisonous, that acute appendicitis can be fatal, and so on. These commonplaces are as familiar to the religious person as to the nonreligious; they are part of the common stock of background information shared within a culture. Hence, the religious risk taker, at least when the risks are understood to be common, physical ones, will have a fair amount of background knowledge about the risks he or she takes. A snake handler knows that rattlesnake bites can be fatal; that is what makes snake handling important and why it serves as a test of faith.[10] Similarly, Faith Assembly members know that hemorrhage in childbirth can be fatal; that is why it is a test of commitment to the church's beliefs to refuse treatment and why, in the controversial case of Sally Burkitt (a Faith Assembly member who bled to death during the delivery of her baby), assisted only by prayer and not by a midwife or physician, Sally pleaded for a doctor instead. Of course, in many cases religious risk takers will not know the precise degree of risk involved (as most of us do not know the precise risk from hemorrhage in childbirth or from untreated rattlesnake bites), but we all share a general conception of the relative dangers of these threats. It is against this background conception of general estimates of danger that religious risk taking occurs.

Yet it is possible to change an individual's estimate of the likelihood that various possible outcomes will occur. Given an array of evaluated possible outcomes, this may involve making specific positively valued outcomes seem more likely or making specific negatively valued ones seem less likely, or both, so that a recalculation of the risk would result in a different choice.

Take, for instance, the case of the Christian Scientist with acute appendicitis who seeks relief. Like other members of contemporary society, he or she will have some background understanding of the likelihood of untreated appendicitis's resulting in death. Although this is by no means a scientifically rigorous conception, the person can say, for instance, that the likelihood of death is greater in untreated appendicitis than in, for example, untreated influenza. However, the teachings of the individual's church persuade him or her that although this background information is accepted by nonbelievers and correctly describes the probabilities confronting them, the probabilities are quite different for persons who understand the nonphysical nature of illness and disease, the power of Christian Science healing, and the true nature of prayer. The believer holds that achieving a correct understanding of "illness" and "disease" as resulting from defective mental attitudes will free him or her from them, even when the risks would otherwise be very high, and that the way to achieve this correct understanding is in prayer. Thus, the Christian Scientist will hold that the risk of death from acute appendicitis treated only with Christian Science prayer is, in fact, much lower than the shared cultural conception would insist; in fact, that it is actually lower not only than the risk from untreated appendicitis but lower than the risk in appendicitis treated with conventional medicine. Prayer, in this view, is the most effective treatment of all. This shared perception of risk explains why Christian Scientists exhibit similar, though unusual, risk budgets in medical choices of this sort; it also invites us to ask how this shared perception of risk is attained.

How does the believing Christian Scientist reach this still lower estimate of the probability of death? Let us look at the kind of evidence with which the believer is supplied and upon which he or she bases prudential calculations of risk; these involve alterations of risk budgets and styles.

Support for claims of the efficacy of Christian Science healing, following the pattern of assertions made in *Science and Health with Key to the Scriptures*[11] and other writings of Mary Baker Eddy, is provided largely by the testimonials of those who recount the ways in which they have been healed from disease or injury. These testimonials are typically quite detailed and fervently sincere in tone; they are direct, firsthand accounts of what is often an extremely powerful, faith-confirming experience. For example, a woman living in the Mojave Desert area of California writes: "On a warm afternoon last May while coming into our house through the laundry room (which is part of the garage), I felt a sharp pain in my right foot. Looking down, I saw what appeared to be a rattlesnake disappearing under the washing machine."[12]

She goes on to recount her fear, the assistance of the Christian Science practitioner in praying for her recovery, the development and eventual subsiding of a discolored, numb swelling on her foot, and the confirming effects this experience had upon her faith.

This testimonial is typical of the handful published in each issue of the *Christian Science Journal,* a monthly periodical widely circulated among Christian Scientists and, like the weekly *Christian Science Sentinel,* a primary source of information about the church. The *Journal* asserts that "the statements made in these testimonies with regard to healings have been carefully verified,"[13] and that it retains on file the originals of testimonials together with the three written verifications or vouchers required for publication. Between 1900 and 1985, some 53,900 testimonials of healing had been published in the periodicals of the church; they are said to be "the most important body of evidence concerning Christian Science healing."[14]

A careful examination of testimonials published in Christian Science periodicals between 1971 and 1981, according to a First Church of Christ, Scientist, authority defending healing in the *New England Journal of Medicine,* shows "647 testimonies concerning illnesses that had been medically diagnosed, in some cases both before and after a healing . . . [including] leukemia and other neoplasias, both malignant and benign; diphtheria; gallstones; pernicious anemia; club feet; spinal meningitis; and bone fracture, among numerous others."[15] This figure includes 137 pediatric cases. Healing in such cases might seem to constitute an impressive record. But the record is wholly anecdotal in form, appealing simply to isolated cases without reference either to general patterns or trends or to comparisons based on control groups. The effect of this kind of information—independently of whether the claims are actually true—is to exacerbate one of the most common errors in decision making under risk.

Many kinds of error are possible in risk-taking choice. Objective errors include misidentification of the range of possible outcomes and assignment of faulty probabilities to possible outcomes (often as the product of subjective factors such as unwarranted optimism or pessimism), misidentification of the values one assigns to possible outcomes, inconsistent weightings of possible outcomes, self-deception, and so on. But there is a common, documentable error characteristic of rational choice, frequently discussed with reference to informed consent in medical situations. This is the tendency to overrely on case information and to underrely on base-rate information.[16] Ordinary patients in ordinary medical contexts do this: They tend to base decisions on anecdotal accounts, supplied by physicians, friends, personal experience, or other sources, including movies and TV, and to downplay or ignore information about the rates of incidence of specific conditions, side effects, self-limiting conditions, spontaneous recovery, and so on.

Whereas ordinary medical patients do this rather naturally, Christian Scientists in situations of medical risk are in effect *encouraged* to do so, since they are supplied with information that makes miscalculation inevitable. What are *not* available from the Christian Science church or from its publications are data that might counteract this tendency or could contribute to establishing reliable base-rate information: How often, given a specific medical condition, does Christian Science healing appear to be effective? This question is much easier to answer than, How often is Christian Science healing actually effective? But no data are available even for the easier question about apparent results.

Clearly, 647 documented cases over a ten-year period is sparse evidence, in view of the number of Scientists and the frequency within the general population of the conditions involved. There might, of course, be many undiagnosed, undocumented cases or a lower incidence of the conditions among the Christian Science population, but these conjectures do little to provide the Christian Scientist with a reliable sense of the frequency with which Christian Science healing, once attempted, is effective. Testimonials of failures, of course, are not published in the church's periodicals.

Yet there is at least some documented information available concerning failures. A study of child fatalities associated with religious groups opposing medical treatment examined the records of 172 children who died between 1975 and 1995 in which there was evidence that parents had withheld medical care because of reliance on religious rituals or teachings and there was sufficient documentation to determine the cause of death.[17] Of the 172 deaths, 140 were from conditions for which survival rates with medical care would have exceeded 90 percent, conditions like pneumonia, meningitis, aspiration, type 1 diabetes, dehydration, diphtheria, measles, appendicitis, and small bowel obstruction. Eighteen more had expected survival rates of over 50 percent. Although this study can be challenged on design grounds, since calculation of overall mortality rates is not possible and the cases were collected in a nonrigorous manner, as the authors recognize, nevertheless the cases do shed light on the importance of negative information. (Interestingly, in this study, Christian Science had a lower number of deaths in proportion to the size of its membership than other groups studied: the Church of the First Born, End Time Ministries, the Faith Assembly, and the Faith Tabernacle.)[18]

Furthermore, the lack of negative information made available to Christian Scientists is compounded by false positives—cases in which Christian Science healing is credited with the cure of a condition that was self-limiting or would have resolved spontaneously anyway—as when the cold that vanishes after troubling a person for two weeks is taken as proof that Christian Science really works.[19] Even the account by the woman bitten by the rattlesnake under her washing machine should be seen in light of the fact that rattlesnake bites are comparatively seldom fatal, especially at distant sites on a limb (the woman was bitten on the foot); but this information was not provided. Yet it is only with adequate base-rate information, making it possible to calculate overall frequencies of success and failure in non-self-limiting conditions with given forms of treatment, that a person can rationally compare conventional medical treatment with Christian Science healing of the same condition, and make a choice in an informed way.[20]

To assert that Christian Science healing cannot be chosen on a rational basis is, of course, not to assume that Christian Science healing is in fact less effective than conventional medical therapy. This point must be conceded by critics of the group, given substantial rates of iatrogenic illness in conventional treatment and the fact that a very large proportion (variously estimated at 75 or 80 percent) of the "illnesses" initially seen by physicians are either self-limiting or psychogenic in origin. Rather, it is to point out that the basis on which a Christian Scientist makes a choice in seeking relief from symptoms is not rationally defensible. Christian Science healing might, in fact, be more effective than conventional medicine, but even the Christian Scientist would have no way of knowing this. Yet the church does claim to supply persuasive, empirical *evidence* for the efficacy of healing; this is part of the point of *Science and Health with Key to the Scriptures* and part of the point of providing testimonials at all.

But the issue is more complicated than it might appear. Nicholas Rescher takes the crucial distinction in risk assessment to be that between *realistic* and *unrealistic* appraisal.[21] Despite the fact that the individual Christian Scientist's choice to rely on Christian Science healing is not rationally defensible, it cannot be said to be unrealistic in a general sense. This is because the individual Scientist has not exaggerated, underestimated, misinterpreted, or otherwise misapprehended or distorted the available evidence. Given the evidence he or she has, the tools provided for assessing it, and the surrounding claim of a trusted institution that the evidence is compelling, he or she makes a subjectively realistic assessment; the fault is not the Scientist's, who is both a believer and a member of the church. In fact, the Christian Scientist characteristically believes that such a choice is a good, sound decision based on a large body of compelling evidence that, though ignored by non-Scientists, is rationally persuasive. As one Scientist wrote:

My own family has relied on Christian Science for generations. I have never considered prayer a gamble. Please understand: I'm not speaking of some crude kind of "faith healing" that implores God to heal and says it was His will if nothing happens. I'm speaking of responsible spiritual healing practiced now over a century by many perfectly normal citizens and caring parents.

I'm concerned about not being taken seriously—that nobody in the media . . . is really taking into account that these healings have been happening over many years. Not just in my family, not just my friends. I'm speaking of the massive, long-term experience in a whole denomination.[22]

If this believer's assessment of risk, although subjectively realistic, is in fact objectively unrealistic, any moral complaint must be directed not primarily against the believer, nor against church teachers and officials, since after all they too share the same set of assumptions with the church membership. Rather, blame rests with the institutional perpetration of the claim that the evidence is valid, and the complaint should point out how the encouragement of belief in the efficacy of healing rather than objective confirmation of it compromises the possibility of autonomous choice. Of course, there is fault on both sides. The medical establishment has been as uninterested in examining alleged Christian Science healings (being generally content to assert that either they were spontaneous recoveries, perhaps associated with the placebo effect, or they were inaccurately diagnosed in the first place) as Christian Science has been to provide well-documented evidence, in particular evidence scrutinized under contrary hypotheses.

But there is a further complexity to the risks Christian Scientists take in choosing healing over conventional medical treatment. Not all healing is successful; some people remain incapacitated, some are sent to Christian Science sanitariums or nursing homes, and some die. Christian Science teaching explains this at least in part as the result of a failure on the part of the patient to understand fully his or her own nature as a spiritual being or to pray adequately for release from incorrect attitudes; the devout Scientist believes that the risk of death from "disease" correctly understood and adequately prayed for is nil. But the Scientist, devout or otherwise, is not encouraged to assess, in making risk-taking choices, how likely it is that he or she will correctly understand and adequately pray for release from the condition. This crucially relevant factor in a prudential risk calculation under these religious assumptions is simply not brought into question or discussed, nor is any evidence bearing on it, anecdotal or otherwise, provided. How often does the explanation of a patient's failure to recover appeal to the claim that the patient failed to pray appropriately or had the wrong attitude? This information too is of great relevance in risk-taking choices, yet it is nowhere forthcoming.

Furthermore (although there is some lack of agreement on this issue)[23] Christian Science generally holds that healing through prayer is incompatible with conventional medical treatment, since prayer consists in achieving an understanding of the nature of disease that contradicts the causal, physicalist assumptions of medicine. Stories abound of people being denied continuation of the services of a Christian Science practitioner if they also enter the care of a physician. Patients who enter Christian Science sanitariums receive care only from nurses who are members of the church and from church practitioners; the nurses are prohibited from doing anything "material" to evaluate or relieve disease and suffering.[24] Thus, although conventional physicians are quick to recognize the psychotherapeutic value of ordinary prayer by the patient, whatever advantages might accrue to the ordinary patient from a combination of medical treatment and religiously supported hope are not available to the Christian Scientist. Rather, the Scientist is forced to make a choice between therapies without knowing whether the chance of survival with both kinds of therapy is better or worse than with only one or the other. Christian Science periodicals do not print testimonials from persons who see doctors as well as healers, any more than they do from persons who see doctors alone.

The institutional practice of altering persons' risk budgets by providing only anecdotal information unaccompanied by base-rate data, as Christian Science does, and by ignoring the incidence of failed cases and of any special conditions that must obtain for the supposed course of action to be effective, fails to satisfy yet a third basic initial criterion for autonomous choice: Not only must it be voluntary and rationally unimpaired, as we've seen, but it must also be adequately informed. It is true that anecdotal information of the kind provided in Christian Science periodicals can be extremely effective in stirring faith and may be of great significance in a person's life. It may well produce a sizable placebo effect. And it is possible that Christian Science healing is actually efficacious, even in cases of non-self-limiting, serious illness. But insofar as merely anecdotal information is put forward as the evidence for claims of efficacy in healing and as a basis for refusing conventional medical treatment, it is clearly an inadequate basis upon which to encourage people to take such substantial risks. Neither their reliance on religious healing nor their refusal of conventional medical treatment meets the conditions for "informed consent." Hence, if we are to assess the practices of this church in the same way we would assess those of medicine or other secular professions that encourage people to take life-threatening risks without granting them the right to give informed consent, we would be tempted to say that they involve manipulation, callousness, or deceit.

The analysis given here of evidentiary claims concerning the efficacy of nonmedical healing applies not only to Christian Science but to any religious group that appeals to alternative varieties of healing, whether the healing involves denominational practitioners, faith healers, or the assumed direct influence of a divine being. The Faith Assembly, for instance, regards Jesus as the sole physician, but (at least if the scant evidence available concerning this group is correct) relies on much the same persuasive structures (where it does not directly coerce) Christian Science uses to produce acceptance of its claim. So do individual faith healers of various sorts, groups such as the Church of the First Born and the Faith Tabernacle Congregation, and many of the contemporary "televangelist" preachers. Methods used to further beliefs about the efficacy of healing at such institutions as the Roman Catholic shrine at Lourdes might also bear inquiry, as well as the practices of groups that accept faith healing but do not reject conventional medical treatment, such as the Assemblies of God and certain charismatic subgroups of Catholicism and Anglicanism. Thus, although Christian Science may provide the most conspicuous example of a certain sort of religious intervention in high-risk decision making, it has many features in common with other groups; ethical censure, if it is appropriate at all, ought hardly be reserved for this group alone.

The Doctrinal Status of Risk Taking

To show that risk-taking religious conduct occurs in various forms and with various amounts of risk in various religious groups—including Christian Science—is not yet to reach a normative conclusion. It cannot simply be assumed that making a decision in which one risks death is wrong, nor can it be assumed that there is something wrong with the mechanisms that religious groups employ to influence people in making these decisions—however extreme the risks, however manipulative the manner of encouraging them, and however severe the consequences for both the risk taker and for others. These are the features that an examination of religious practices using professional ethics exposes; yet to identify features is not to establish that they are morally intolerable, since such conduct is governed not only by moral considerations but also by the doctrines, teachings, and authoritative pronouncements of the specific religious groups.

In my volume *Ethics in the Sanctuary,* I developed a typology to distinguish various levels of doctrinal assertions with respect to the ethical dilemmas involved.[25] The typology recognizes four distinct levels or orders of doctrinal assertions: 0-order or base-level doctrines, the fundamental imperatives of a group (often, though not always, stated in scriptural texts); first-order doctrines or teachings, which stipulate ways of putting basic imperatives into practice but characteristically generate new moral problems in doing so; second-order doctrines or teachings, which establish a position that attempts to resolve the ethical problems presented by first-order doctrines; and third-order doctrines or teachings, which function as excuses for residual moral problems. This four-level typology provides a basis for distinguishing the more fundamental religious imperatives of a group from dictates that, though they may have achieved similar doctrinal status, exhibit later historical or theoretical development within a tradition and are best viewed as "answers" to and "excuses" for the moral problems posed by the fundamental imperatives and the ways they are put into practice. Because of their derivative status, whatever doctrinal position they may enjoy, they are to be treated as initially more vulnerable to ethical review than the basic imperatives of the tradition within which they arise.

In surveying the huge variety of risk-taking practices evident among various Christian and Christian-influenced groups, this typology serves to differentiate between those risk-taking dictates that are more vulnerable and those that are less vulnerable to ethical criticism. Of course, since the risk-taking practices in these groups—including Christian Science—do not form a coherent, unified, single tradition but occur in a spectrum of denominations and sects with different histories, application of this typology will not be completely tidy or uniform. Nevertheless, it is possible to identify doctrines, directives, teachings, and other authoritative pronouncements at all four levels.

In these religious settings, some people take risks, including physical risks, and some of these risks eventuate badly: some persons suffer serious damage to their health; some die. The topology employed here reveals a further level of doctrinal, quasi-doctrinal, or authoritative claim, identified as third-order doctrine, that provides "excuses" for the residual moral problems generated by the practices in question. For instance, when a Christian Scientist practicing his or her beliefs by relying on healing refuses conventional medical treatment and dies, some account consistent with both the basic doctrinal imperative and with the first- and second-order teachings is needed to explain or justify the negative outcome.

Similarly, since serpent handlers act to honor the assertion in Mark 16 that "they will pick up snakes in their hands, and if they drink any deadly thing, it will not hurt them," the group's continued acceptance of the basic religious imperative depends in part on providing a doctrinally acceptable account of how snake bites and snake bite fatalities can occur, that is, an excuse for the negative outcome resulting from the risks a person takes in relying on the scriptural assurance that no harm will come from handling snakes.

These third-order teachings or excuses for failed risks are usually easy to identify, though they are not always encoded in official doctrine. When a Christian Scientist who refuses medical treatment and relies on prayer worsens or dies, the most frequent explanation is that he or she failed to pray adequately and hence failed to achieve the proper understanding of the nature of disease. Similarly, the Faith Assembly member who dies after refusing treatment is said to have lacked faith in Jesus' power to heal—an accusation so prevalent in this group that its founder, Hobart Freeman, extended it even to those who use automobile seat belts. The serpent handler who is bitten is sometimes said to have failed to be sure of being genuinely anointed before taking up the snakes.

Just as it is easy to identify these third-order teachings or excuses for the negative outcomes that a group's risk-taking practices have brought about, it is also easy to see a feature that is common to many of them: They explain the negative outcome as a result of a failure on the part of the individual harmed. This is true in the Faith Assembly, the Holiness Church, and Christian Science. In examining the excuses various groups encode in their doctrines, we can begin by considering whether excuses that lay the blame for unsuccessful risk taking at the feet of the risk taker are themselves morally defensible, or whether a defensible excuse must be of some other form.

In contrast, the Jehovah's Witnesses appear to offer no excuse when a Witness refuses transfusion and dies. However, under the reevaluation that is characteristic of Jehovah's Witness practice, there is nothing to excuse. The faithful Witness who dies because he or she refuses blood—according to the teachings of the group—nevertheless achieves salvation, which, under the reevaluation, is the maximally valued outcome the choice could yield. Consequently, for the devout, the death need not be excused. The issue, then, is whether Christian Science is like this, or whether Christian Science involves a pragmatic attempt to achieve cure: Does Christian Science involve praying for a cure, or praying for its own sake, believing—but not centrally intending—that this might also result in cure?

The Moral Evaluation of Risk Taking in Religion

Examining the practices of Christian Science and other groups suggests an immediate conclusion: that these practices involving risks cannot be morally defended, and, furthermore, that they should be denounced on moral grounds. In *Ethics in the Sanctuary,* I argue that the developed practices and teachings of religious groups, as distinct from their fundamental imperatives, are vulnerable to ethical critique. And when we now look at these practices in a variety of groups, including Christian Science, we see that they involve clear abuses of identifiable, uncontroversial moral principle. Examining issues in confidentiality in many groups, for example, Catholics, Mormons, and fundamentalist groups like the Collinsville Church of Christ, we find practices that variously involve lying, nonconsenting disclosure, manipulation, and allowing serious, preventable harms.[26] Thus risk taking in a variety of groups involves coercion, impairment of rational capacities, manipulation, callousness, and deception. No doubt we could look further and find more. But to identify these apparent moral abuses is not to establish that they are abuses *in religious contexts;* we have only seen them this way because we instinctively appeal to principles familiar in secular life. Even though we have established that certain religious doctrines and practices are open to ethical evaluation, we cannot simply assume that the principles presupposed by this catalogue of apparent abuses are applicable here.

Of the moral principles that these apparent abuses seem to violate, autonomy is central. This principle is highlighted by the strategy of using the apparatus of professional ethics to examine issues of religious risk taking, in particular, the concept of informed consent. The principle of autonomy, received in both its Kantian form and in the utilitarian version defended by John Stuart Mill, is seldom contested in either ordinary or professional ethics, though there certainly are continuing, vigorous debates about how it should be interpreted, about the degree to which individuals are capable of genuine autonomy, and about when, if ever, the principle may be overridden. This principle has been central in contemporary professional ethics. Here too disagreement virtually or nearly exclusively concerns the conditions under which paternalistic or harm-based exceptions to the principle are legitimate; there are few real challenges to the principle of autonomy itself.

Do these religious practices violate the principle of autonomy and thus undercut the possibility of informed consent? Though they are often explicated within professional ethics in more elaborate ways, the conditions for autonomous choice involve three criteria: (1) the decision must be uncoerced, (2) it must be rationally unimpaired, and (3) it must be adequately informed. But, as we have seen, these are precisely the conditions that the practices of these various groups violate.[27] The Faith Assembly, at least on some occasions, coerces its members into refusing medical treatment. The Holiness serpent-handling groups encourage making potentially fatal decisions about handling snakes under extreme emotional impairment, calling that condition an "anointment" for taking the risk. Christian Science provides selective, anecdotal information only, without base or failure rates, in a way that is inevitably deceptive in influencing a high-risk choice. Nor is it apparent that these interferences in autonomous choice can be excused on the ground of limiting risks to third parties or for compelling paternalist reasons. Thus, since these practices are vulnerable to ethical critique and the infractions of the principle of autonomy are so clear, it would seem that moral conclusions could be drawn readily.

But I do not think this is so. Because our apparatus for evaluating religious practice is not yet complete, the principle of autonomy cannot be directly employed. Upper-level doctrines and practices are *candidates* for critique; but we have yet to establish on what basis the critique can be made. To condemn practices for violating conditions of autonomous choice involves an unwarranted leap in ethical evaluation, even though these criteria are well established in both professional and ordinary ethics. It is a leap we can make—in limited ways—only after our initial typology is supplemented with the appropriate critical principle.

The principle to which we shall appeal, the fiduciary principle, is a distinct moral principle not reducible either to that of autonomy or to those of nonmaleficence and beneficence. Most explicitly articulated in law, it is vaguely recognized in various forms in all of the secular professions. The fiduciary principle serves to identify the obligations of the professional vis-à-vis the client in professional contexts and, except for a few distinctive interpersonal relationships, it is usually thought to be limited to professional contexts.

To employ a principle adopted from professional ethics to examine organized religion is not to presuppose that religious functionaries are all professionals in the fullest sense. Clergy of the mainstream denominations have traditionally been regarded in this way, though cult leaders, evangelists, faith healers, gurus, and the like have not. Although the fiduciary principle has been developed in professional contexts, its scope is broader and provides a crucial distinction in assessing religious practice.

The fiduciary principle, which applies to all aspects of professional-client interaction, regulates practice by stipulating that it must be possible for the client to *trust* the professional in the course of the interaction, even though the professional's own interests may conflict with those of the client. Put another way, the fiduciary principle prohibits the professional from taking advantage of the client—violating the client's rights or harming his or her interests—in the course of the professional relationship, though the professional's superior status, power, and knowledge would make it easy to do so. For example, the lawyer has fiduciary duties to the client; this means that the lawyer must use his or her professional skills to advance the client's interests or, at least, not to harm them. Similarly, the trustee, as fiduciary to the beneficiary of a trust fund, must refrain from usurping the beneficiary's interests in the fund, just as the director of a corporation must refrain from promoting his or her own interests at the expense of the corporation. The fiduciary principle may seem similar to the more general principle of nonmaleficence, but it has a specific application to the professional-client relationship and to the characteristic imbalance of power this relationship exhibits. It is broader in scope than the comparatively narrow principle of autonomy; it requires the professional not only to respect the client's autonomous choices and to protect the client's capacity to make them but also to ensure (and this does not rule out paternalistic intervention) that the client's interests are served. Thus, the principle is a complex one, with conditions often in tension between autonomist and paternalist demands, and it is not reducible to the simpler principles often cited in professional and ordinary moral discourse. To say, as Charles Fried does, that the fiduciary "owes a duty of strict and unreserved loyalty to his client"[28] is correct and makes it clear that the professional's primary obligation is to the client, not the professional's own interests, the institution, or others who might be involved. But the question of how the sometimes conflicting requirements of this complex principle are to be satisfied is left open.

Inasmuch as the fiduciary principle has autonomist components, the three conditions for the protection of autonomous choice identified above—noncoercion, freedom from rational impairment, and adequate informedness—can all be derived from it, though in some circumstances they may be in tension with paternalist components of the principle. In professional areas such as medicine and law, these three conditions protect the client from the professional in very specific ways. The client, it is assumed, consults the professional in order to advance his or her aims and interests; the protection needed is protection from possible dishonesty, manipulation, or greed on the part of the professional. For instance, when the patient consults the doctor for help in curing an illness, he or she occupies an unequal, vulnerable position in the relationship (the patient, after all, is both sick and untrained in medicine) and must rely on the physician's obligations as fiduciary to keep from being made worse off, specifically, from being made worse off with respect to health. The legal client consults an attorney for help in protecting his or her rights and similarly relies on the attorney's fiduciary obligation to a client. Since the attorney is far more skilled in the law than the client, the attorney could easily jeopardize the client's rights. Professionals are also often in a position to jeopardize other interests of the client (both doctors and lawyers, for instance, can easily threaten a patient's or client's emotional, social, or financial well-being), but it is with respect to the specific interest or set of interests about which the client has consulted the professional that the fiduciary principle most directly applies.

Like other professionals, the religious professional, whether minister, priest, rabbi, pastor, evangelist, faith healer, or guru, is in a position to make individuals within the group either better or worse off. He or she can affect their emotional, social, financial, or other peripheral interests. The religious professional can also affect, either positively or negatively, the specific aim or interest for which they seek help in the first place; it is this fact that initially supports the appeal to the fiduciary principle made here. What the fiduciary principle requires is that the priest or the preacher not treat those who come as prey, even in the most subtle ways, or use them either for self-interested ends or other institutional goals but instead remain worthy of trust.

To construe the relation between the religious professional and member of the religious group in this way invites us to identify precisely what it is that the religious believer comes to the religious professional for, that is, what interests he or she hopes to serve in approaching the religious professional. Although this may be very difficult to do for a specific case, we can venture certain general observations. Consider, for instance, the reasons why the Christian Scientist or a member of the Faith Assembly has contact with the leaders of his or her group, as contrasted with the reasons why, for example, a member of a serpent-handling group might do so. The Christian Scientist calls a practitioner when he or she is ill and does so for help in restoring health. Similarly, the member of the Faith Assembly rejects medicine and relies on Jesus in order to get well, but he or she also acts to retain membership and avoid humiliation by the group. The serpent handler, on the other hand, attends a prayer meeting and handles serpents in order to satisfy the injunction he or she believes Mark 16 states; there is less evidence here of some particular external objective. Then again, the Jehovah's Witness appears to refuse blood in order to satisfy a biblical commandment, much as the serpent handler does, but does so in order not to jeopardize his or her chances of salvation.

Of course, identifying reasons why people engage in religion is a murky business at best; a full psychological explanation of such behaviors is far more complex than can be treated here. Nevertheless, it is evident that strikingly different degrees of rational prudence, in the pursuit of self-interest, are exhibited by the members of various groups. The Christian Scientist seeks to get well, just as any ordinary patient seeing any ordinary doctor does; in doing so, the Scientist acts to promote one of his or her interests—health. The Scientist does not call the condition "illness" nor recognize its symptoms as those of "disease," nor does he or she understand the end state sought to be a "cure" but rather a "demonstration" of the truth of the principles of Christian Science. Indeed, the Scientist rejects the entire causal metaphysics of medicine. Nevertheless, he or she accepts, and the church promotes, a variety of external similarities, many dating from the earliest period of the church,[29] reinforcing the claim that what the believer seeks is what any ordinary patient seeks: help in regaining health. For instance, the Christian Scientist calls the practitioner only when he or she has discomforting symptoms (whether or not viewed as symptoms of "disease"). The practitioner can be found by looking in the Yellow Pages; an appointment is made; the practitioner's services are paid for at rates roughly comparable to those of a physician; and, in some states (Massachusetts, for instance) Blue Cross will pay the bill. To put it another way, Christian Science functions as an alternative health care system, though it denies medicine's metaphysics and makes no use of medical techniques; we can easily identify the professional institution to which Christian Science promotes itself as an alternative. But in doing so, the way in which Christian Science encourages risk taking is different from that of many other religious groups.

Not all risk-taking practices function as alternatives to secular professional institutions. The serpent handler, for example, does not so clearly seek to advance his or her interests by risking health or life but instead acts simply to obey an injunction he or she believes is what the Lord demands. There do not seem to be external similarities promoted by the group that would reinforce the claim that in handling snakes the believer attempts to further the same aims and interests that clients of other professionals do. Serpent handling is not an *alternative* anything; it is simply a practice of the group.

Noting these differences should allow us to see why the fiduciary principle, although vaguely asserted in the secular professions, is not discussed much there and why, in contrast, it is of particular interest in the religious sphere. The fiduciary principle prohibits the professional from violating moral principles in a way that would undermine those aims or interests for which a client seeks protection or advancement in using the professional's services. In medicine and law, as in other secular professions, this covers the entire range of cases: Patients and legal clients use the services of doctors and lawyers in order to protect and advance their own aims or interests, or those of organizations and causes with which they identify, and generally not for any other reason. They come to lawyers and doctors to protect their rights, broadly construed, or to get well. Since virtually all of the activities in which the professional engages with the client are initiated in response to such purposes on the part of the client, there is nothing distinctive in these areas of professional practice that the fiduciary principle might isolate and identify as protected under this principle. Of course, some clients do not voluntarily consult professionals but are delivered to them, such as the unconscious emergency patient or the impoverished defendant in the criminal justice system. But even in these circumstances the fiduciary principle applies by extension. On some occasions a client might consult a professional for purposes that do not appear to serve his or her self-interests, as, for example, when a person consults a doctor to donate a kidney to someone else. But even here the patient does so with the aim of protecting his or her interests as well as those of the recipient and does not ask the doctor to remove the kidney without regard for his or her own health. Even if the fiduciary principle is not particularly conspicuous in the secular professions, largely because it covers virtually all available cases, it will nevertheless play a central role in sorting out those cases in religion to which ordinary moral norms apply and those to which they do not.

The fiduciary principle functions in critiquing religious practice by identifying under what conditions upper-level practices and doctrines may be reviewed with the moral principles available in professional and ordinary ethics—such principles as autonomy, nonmaleficence, and beneficence. Although the working typology employed earlier makes it possible to distinguish between fundamental, 0-level imperatives and upper-level, developed doctrines and practices, it does not specify whether all of the latter are actually open to critique. The fiduciary principle functions as a second general principle, supplementing the earlier typology, and further limits the application of moral norms to religious practices. The fiduciary principle itself does not aid in sorting out conflicts and tensions between the demands of autonomy, nonmaleficence, and beneficence, either in general or in specific cases; this is work for the applied professional ethicist concerned with organized religion, the "ecclesioethicist," to do. But the principle does tell us when the ecclesioethicist can get to work, by telling us under what conditions the basic moral principles can be applied to upper-level doctrines and practices. In religious contexts, the fiduciary principle asserts that *the developed practices, doctrines, methods, and teachings employed by religious professionals or their religious organizations must meet (secular) ethical criteria wherever the individual participates in these practices to advance his or her self-interests.* The fact that the religious professional is *religious* does not exempt him or her from treating clients in ways that are morally binding in the secular professions, as well as in ordinary morality, whenever the client approaches the religious professional for the same sorts of self-interest-serving purposes for which he or she would approach a secular professional—even if the client is also a believer and adherent of the group. For example, if the Christian Scientist seeks help from a Christian Scientist practitioner *in order to get well,* then he or she is entitled to the same freedom from coercion, from impairment, and to the same adequate information to which an ordinary medical patient would be entitled in seeking to get well. In a word, the religious believer, like the medical patient, is entitled to the protections of informed consent; the believer's status as a believer does not abrogate this right. However, if a believer approaches a Christian Science practitioner not to get well but in order to deepen his or her faith, as many devout Christian Scientists clearly do, then it is not so clear that these constraints apply. Many Christian Scientists conceive of healing not as an alternative medical system at all but as a process of prayer that is part of the effort to achieve a certain spiritual condition. A side effect of that process, though not its central purpose, may be the restoration of health.[30] It is indeed crucial whether the Christian Scientist is praying *for a cure* or praying for the sake of praying, though believing that cure may also result.

It may seem that the religious organization, or the religious professional within it, can have no such fiduciary obligation, inasmuch as neither the professional nor the organization has control over the reasons for which an individual approaches them. This is not so, of course, for the way in which a religious organization, including its officials, is approached is very much a function of the way in which it announces or advertises itself. After all, announcing or advertising an organization is an interactive process between the organization and the individuals who approach it. The process is not much remarked upon in the secular professions, since most secular professions announce themselves in uniform ways, but it is a process of

tremendous variability in religion. Christian Science, for instance, announces and promotes itself as an alternative healing system by the very fact
that it distributes testimonials that recount favorable recoveries using
Christian Science healing (even though these testimonials are described
primarily as serving to give thanks to God) and by asking Blue Cross to
cover the services it renders. In response to the way in which Christian Science announces and promotes itself, prospective users of the church
approach it in kind, seeking to receive these services in order to further
their aims and interests in getting well. The fact that prospective users of
Christian Science healing, both members and prospective converts, seek to
further their aims and interests in getting well leads the church and its officials to promote the church's services in this way. Similarly, for example,
the Church of Scientology promotes itself as providing help in achieving
psychological stability and growth; in this sense, it attempts to function as
an alternative psychotherapeutic profession. As in Christian Science, Scientology's public stance is interactive with the aims and purposes for which
prospective users of its services approach the church: It announces itself as
able to provide psychological help and personality development, and people who seek these things turn to it.

In the secular professions, when we talk about a client's reasons for seeking a professional, we are saying as much about the professional and the
background organization as we are about the client. Thus, to phrase the
fiduciary principle in terms of what the client seeks is also to identify specific professional and institutional postures. In religion, since the fiduciary
principle underwrites the application of standard ethical principles (for
example, the bioethics canon of autonomy, nonmaleficence, beneficence,
and justice) when adherents approach with self-interested aims, it thus also
underwrites the application of these principles when the religious group
and its officials announce themselves as available to help persons pursue
their interests.

Of course, virtually all religious invitation may contain some appeal to
self-interest. Insofar as a group makes such an invitation, however, under
the interpretation of the fiduciary principle advanced here, it is obligated
to protect and promote the aims and self-interests to which the invitation
is directed. The church that announces itself as able to satisfy certain interests of persons who are attracted to the church in this way opens itself
to *secular* moral critique of the practices and doctrines it employs in satis-
fying those interests. Not all of the upper-order practices in a religious
group will be susceptible to ethical critique under the fiduciary principle;
but many of those that have been traditionally protected by the notion of

religious immunity will be clear targets for ethical examination and can be assessed using the secular moral criteria developed in ordinary and professional ethics. (Curiously, the distinction between upper-level practices that are vulnerable to ethical critique and those that are not is reflected, though somewhat crudely, in the growing area of clergy malpractice insurance. Malpractice insurance is available in approximately those areas in which clergy do what other professionals do, especially counseling, but not for practices much less directly related to the satisfaction of individual self-interests, such as the performance of rites, the maintenance of beliefs, or the upholding of orthodoxy.) The distinction is not always clear; most groups give off mixed signals and are approached for mixed reasons. Nevertheless, the theoretical importance of this distinction is considerable.

I began with a discussion of the practices of various religious groups in encouraging their adherents to take risks, focusing particularly on Christian Science. In this discussion, appeal has been made to both general moral principles, such as autonomy, nonmaleficence, beneficence, and justice, and to their application in requirements such as informed consent. I argued that upper-level practices such as these, which encourage risk, are candidates for moral critique, but I did not demonstrate why critique is appropriate in these specific cases. Use of the fiduciary principle provides an answer. At least in the case of the Christian Science, Jehovah's Witnesses, and the Holiness churches, there is good reason to think that individuals consult religious professionals to promote their own interests and that these groups promote characteristic practices under a corresponding appeal to self-interest of the members of the group. Christian Scientists choose prayer over medicine in order to get well; the church promotes prayer as a means of healing. The Jehovah's Witnesses refuse blood to avoid precluding salvation; this church and its officials promote the practice of refusing blood at least in part with this rationale. If it turns out that the serpent handler does not act to obey the biblical commandment but simply seeks the heightened sensory or emotional experience provided by the dangerous thrill of handling snakes, then this too belongs under ordinary ethical scrutiny. After all, heightened sensory or emotional experience is available in ways that are less life threatening.

Applications of the fiduciary principle in organized religion are not likely to be easy in practice. The principle refers to the reasons for which people use religious services, as induced by the religious organization and vice versa, and these reasons may be multifarious and obscure. Nor can we assume that the reasons for which people consult religious professionals are as uniform as the reasons for which they consult doctors or lawyers.

Individuals go to church or see their ministers for an enormous variety of reasons, including relieving anxiety, coping with fear, preserving a marriage, restoring health, increasing security, dealing with grief, curbing aggressive or suicidal impulses, maintaining social standing, and so on. A very large part of what leads the religious believer to a religious professional involves the protection and advancement of interests like these; a very large part of the comforts that religious groups offer are directed toward the satisfaction of these interests. Self-interested religious behavior may be very difficult to distinguish from self-interested nonreligious behavior. However cumbersome applications of the principle might be in practice and, consequently, however poor a basis it might make for policy formation, it is an appropriate basis for distinguishing those religious activities and practices that are proper targets for ethical critique from those that are comparatively immune.

It is also a proper basis for scrutinizing the way that religious groups advertise themselves and their services, both in securing continuing commitment from their members and in attracting new ones. The televangelist groups and their leaders are particularly revealing targets for scrutiny. Oral Roberts, for example, makes a direct appeal to the financial interests of prospective contributors by promising immediate material reward. Roberts has sent multicolored prayer sheets to his "prayer partners" to be mailed back (together with a contribution) with a list of needs for which he can pray: "The RED area is for your SPIRITUAL healing; the WHITE area is for your PHYSICAL healing; the GREEN area is for your FINANCIAL healing. Check the needs you have and RUSH them back to me."[31] Roberts is by no means the only media preacher who announces his brand of religion as likely to enhance a believer's interests in material comfort and financial success. But because televangelists invite persons to approach them for the same sorts of reasons for which they might approach a secular financial counselor or investment firm, they are open to the same sort of ethical critique. In general, religious operatives promising satisfaction of their audience's financial interests provide a ripe field for further inquiry.

However, not all individuals approach religious professionals or organizations to promote their own self-interests. Consider, for instance, the person who sees a minister or goes to church in order to "strengthen my faith." This seemingly central religious purpose bears close scrutiny, for it must be asked why the believer wants to strengthen this faith. If, for instance, it is evident that the believer seeks assistance in strengthening faith to "be sure to go to heaven," the motive sounds very much like the kind of self-interest that other forms of rational prudence display. Once it is assumed or believed that there is a heaven, then it is not so much a matter of *religion* to want to get there; it is a matter of rational prudence, especially if the only available alternative under this particular belief system is hell. Consequently, even the apparently religious purpose of strengthening one's faith in consulting a religious professional or participating in religious practices falls under the fiduciary principle just articulated. Hence, the professional's methods of providing these services and the established church practices that support them are subject to the same working moral criteria as other areas of professional ethics, at least if we assume that the religious professional is in any way capable of either advancing or undermining the interests a person seeks to advance.

This conclusion does not mean, however, that the same local principles or rules of professional ethics apply in religion as they do in medicine or law. Although the fiduciary principle may provide a basic moral standard for all areas of professional practice, including organized religion, it may be that specific applications of the principles derived from it, as well as local rules such as confidentiality and truth telling, differ from one area of professional practice to another. Thus, for example, principles governing the protection of autonomy in decision making under risk may differ from psychiatry to medicine to sports coaching to religion, but they must all satisfy the general fiduciary requirement that the professional be loyal to the client and not take advantage of him or her.

Although having one's faith strengthened in order to get to heaven may not be a distinctively religious purpose for consulting a religious professional, some purposes are. A person who initially expresses a desire for help in strengthening faith might explain that she seeks this help because God is supremely worthy of worship and therefore she wishes to worship God more fully—regardless of the impact this fuller worship might have on her. This kind of purpose in seeking assistance from a religious professional does not involve seeking to advance one's own interests, thereby putting oneself in a position vulnerable to the professional's influence. Consequently, it is not a purpose to which the usual strictures of professional morality under the fiduciary principle apply. For instance, some Christian Scientists, as perhaps some Faith Assembly members, Jehovah's Witnesses, Holiness Church members, members of the Church of the First Born, End Time Ministries, Faith Tabernacle, or others, may observe their church's teaching not to enhance their health or to secure salvation but simply because they believe it to be the word of God. As yet, we have no basis for applying secular moral criteria in cases like these, regardless of the nature of these practices and doctrines that have developed or the group's methods in promoting this behavior. (This is not, of course, to say that they are justified.) However, these cases may be very few, and such people as rare as saints. If most religious behavior is actually the pursuit of self-interest under a special set of metaphysical assumptions, then the "professionals" who are the purveyors and caretakers of these assumptions in the form of religious doctrine, teachings, and practices are obligated, as in any fiduciary relationship, to protect persons in that pursuit. Christian Science is no exception.

Notes

1. This chapter is drawn from my book *Ethics in the Sanctuary: Examining the Practices of Organized Religion* (New Haven: Yale University Press, 1990). In this book, chapter 2, "High-Risk Religion: Informed Consent in Faith Healing, Serpent Handling, and Refusing Medical Treatment," originally dealt with four high-risk groups: Christian Science, Jehovah's Witnesses, the Faith Assembly, and the Holiness churches. Several additional groups are covered in Seth M. Asser and Rita Swan, "Child Fatalities from Religion-Motivated Medical Neglect," *Pediatrics* 101, no. 4 (April 1998): 625–629.

2. Charles Fried, *An Anatomy of Values: Problems of Personal and Social Choice* (Cambridge: Harvard University Press, 1970), 167.

3. See Thomas C. Johnsen, "Christian Scientists and the Medical Profession: A Historical Perspective," *Medical Heritage* (January–February 1986): 70–78, for a loyal account of the historical background; also see Robert Peel, *Spiritual Healing in a Scientific Age* (San Francisco: Harper & Row, 1987), for a loyal attempt to address scientific issues.

4. Arnold S. Relman, M.D., "Christian Science and the Care of Children," *New England Journal of Medicine* 309, no. 26 (December 29, 1983): 1639.

5. Nathan A. Talbot, "The Position of the Christian Science Church," *New England Journal of Medicine* 309, no. 26 (December 29, 1983): 1641–1644, esp. 1642.

6. Talbot, "Position of the Christian Science Church," 1642.

7. On the distinction between mechanical procedures and other medical treatment, see Arthur E. Nudelman, "The Maintenance of Christian Science in Scientific Society," in *Marginal Medicine,* ed. Roy Wallis and Peter Morley (New York: Free Press, 1976), 42–60; also see William E. Laur, M.D., "Christian Science Visited," *Southern Medical Journal* 73, no. 1 (January 1980): 71–74, esp. 73.

8. Rita Swan, "Faith Healing, Christian Science, and the Medical Care of Children," *New England Journal of Medicine* 309, no. 26 (December 29, 1983): 1640.

9. Also listed in the *Christian Science Journal* are churches, reading rooms, and Christian Science colleges and university organizations. Christian Science care facilities are not listed in the *Journal* but do advertise in church publications.

10. Members of the Holiness churches insist that serpent handling is not to be understood as a "test of faith" in the sense that reciting a creed might be but as a "confirmation" of God's word. Glossolalia, serpent handling, strychnine drinking, and similar practices are the "signs following" belief in God but are not evidence for it. See Robert W. Pelton and Karen W. Carden, *Snake-Handlers: God-Fearers?*

or Fanatics? (Nashville: Thomas Nelson, 1974), which provides a useful pictorial essay on these practices.

11. Mary Baker Eddy, *Science and Health with Key to the Scriptures* (1875; Boston: The First Church of Christ, Scientist, 1934).

12. Merrily Allen Ozengher, *Christian Science Journal* 101, no. 9 (September 1983).

13. A footnote that appears at the beginning of "On Christian Science Healing," a section of testimonials in each issue of the *Christian Science Journal.*

14. Talbot, "Position of the Christian Science Church," 1642; see also *A Century of Christian Science Healing* (Boston: The Christian Science Publishing Society, 1966) for the church's account of this history. The figure is from the Committee on Publication's 1989 paper "An Empirical Analysis of Medical Evidence in Christian Science Testimonies of Healing, 1969–1988," First Church of Christ, Scientist, 175 Huntington Avenue, Boston, Mass. 02115.

15. Talbot, "Position of the Christian Science Church," 1642.

16. See, e.g., Daniel Kahneman, Paul Slovic, and Amos Tversky, eds., *Judgment under Uncertainty: Heuristics and Biases* (Cambridge: Cambridge University Press, 1982).

17. Seth M. Asser and Rita Swan, "Child Fatalities from Religion-Motivated Medical Neglect," *Pediatrics* 101, no. 4 (April 1998): 625–629.

18. Asser and Swan, "Child Fatalities," 628, table 4.

19. Nudelman, "Maintenance of Christian Science in a Scientific Society," 49.

20. Base-rate and related information could presumably be accumulated if Christian Scientists as well as non-Scientists were routinely examined and diagnosed by physicians and if medical records of all procedures (as well as records of healing by prayer) were kept. Of course, this is not generally the case. Neither could the kind of persuasive evidence supplied by controlled clinical trials be obtained on the efficacy of Christian Science healing, since it would not be possible to *randomize* subjects into groups, one of which would (sincerely) perform Christian Science prayer while the other would not pray but would have confidence in conventional medicine alone. The closest approximation to designing such a trial would be (1) to randomize believing Scientists into groups that use prayer and those that, denied the services of a Christian Science practitioner, are offered only conventional treatment or (2) to randomize nonbelievers into those who use conventional medical treatment and those who go through the motions of prayer.

A study cited in the *Hastings Center Report* 19, no. 3 (May–June 1989): 2–3, reports a randomized, double-blind study of the effects of intercessory prayer on hospitalized patients ("Positive Therapeutic Effects of Intercessory Prayer in a Coronary Care Unit Population," *Southern Medical Journal* 81, no. 7 [1988]: 826–829). This study randomized patients who were prayed for by others, not patients who prayed for themselves; nevertheless, it did conclude that the prayed-for group exhibited fewer complications than the control group.

21. Nicholas Rescher, *Risk: A Philosophical Introduction to the Theory of Risk Evaluation and Management* (Washington, D.C.: University Press of America, 1983), 132.

22. Lois O'Brien, "Prayer's Not a Gamble," letter in *U.S. News & World Report,* April 28, 1986, 81.

23. Contrast the symposium articles in the *New England Journal of Medicine* 310, no. 19 (May 10, 1984): 1257–1260, with subsequent letters to the editor.

24. Rita Swan, letter to the editor, *New England Journal of Medicine* 310, no. 19 (May 20, 1984): 1260. Swan is the president of CHILD (Children's Healthcare Is a Legal Duty), a group that opposes exempting Christian Science from obligations to provide medical care for children.

25. I develop the typology over the course of several chapters, including the one from which this essay is drawn. Also see the commentary by Michael Steel, "Religious Practice, Divine Discourse, and Applied Ethics," thesis, Australian Catholic University.

26. The issue of confidentiality and the practices of these groups are discussed in chapter 1 of *Ethics in the Sanctuary.*

27. These explorations are conducted more fully in *Ethics in the Sanctuary,* chapter 2.

28. Charles Fried, *Medical Experimentation, Personal Integrity and Social Policy* (New York: American Elsevier, 1974), 33.

29. By the turn of the century, the medical establishment viewed Christian Science as an alternative (and bogus) school of medicine, not a religion. See Johnsen, "Christian Scientists and the Medical Profession," 72.

30. Johnsen, "Christian Scientists and the Medical Profession," 73. As Johnsen also notes, in 1898 a unanimous opinion of the Rhode Island Supreme Court affirmed that prayer in Christian Science could not be mistaken for the practice of medicine in any "ordinary sense and meaning" of the term.

31. Alan Brinkley, "The Oral Majority," *New Republic,* September 29, 1986, 31.

2

Rational Choice and Alternative Worldviews: A Defense of Christian Science

Peggy DesAutels

The health-related choices made by Christian Scientists are often criticized as being irrational. It is difficult for those who are medically oriented to understand how Christian Scientists can rationally justify avoiding medical treatments that are known to be effective. What is especially confusing to the observer of such choices is that Christian Scientists are, for the most part, well educated and otherwise rational individuals. In this chapter, I analyze the nature of the choices made by Christian Scientists and argue that such choices are neither irrational nor the result of unethical church practices.

In chapter 1, Margaret P. Battin maintains that Christian Science institutional practices result in a Christian Scientist's inability to make an autonomous and informed rational choice when faced with a life-threatening illness or injury. I respond here to Battin's criticisms of Christian Science and argue the following:

1. The Christian Scientist's decision to pursue spiritual means for treatment does not resemble in structure the calculation of risk found in medical decision making, and therefore base-rate information on success rates for healing a particular disease is inapplicable.
2. The Christian Science institutional practice of publishing only accounts of healing successes does not equate to an unethical encouragement of Christian Scientists to make choices from an inadequate basis; rather, the recounting of healings is an integral part of Christian Science worship and is instructional to other Christian Scientists

37

on how to achieve a mental state that, when achieved, always results in both spiritual advancement and physical healing.

3. The primary choice a Christian Scientist makes is not ultimately one of choosing between alternative health care regimes; rather, it is one of choosing between very different worldviews. Making such a choice is more a matter of conscience than of pure rationality.

Battin's Critique of Christian Science Practices

Margaret P. Battin's main criticism of the Christian Science Church is that it fails to provide base-rate and other relevant information on the effectiveness of Christian Science in healing specific medical conditions. As a result, adherents are unable to make a rational choice between a medical approach to healing and a spiritual one. Battin's criticism rests on the view that a health-related choice made by a Christian Scientist resembles in structure any other prudential calculation under risk:

> The choice to accept treatment from a Christian Science practitioner rather than a medical doctor, or not to accept treatment at all, resembles in structure any other prudential calculation under risk: Various possible outcomes— cure, continuing illness, incapacitation, and death—are foreseen under specific valuations and under more or less quantifiable expectations about the likelihood of their occurrence.[1]

In her view, just as the decision of which alternative medical approach to take should be based on the success rates of each medical alternative, so the decision of whether to use a Christian Science approach or a medical approach should be based on the success rates for curing that particular condition using Christian Science and the success rates of each of the medical alternatives. Although the Christian Science Church has published a large body of anecdotal evidence for the successful healing of physical conditions, many of which were medically diagnosed, Battin claims that when Christian Scientists are supplied with such anecdotes without accompanying anecdotes of failure, they are encouraged by their church to miscalculate the risks involved in choosing a Christian Science approach. Battin holds the view shared by many philosophers of science that anecdotal evidence is a much less rational basis for decision making than is base-rate information or experimental evidence that makes use of control groups.

As Battin continues with her analysis of the rationality of a Christian Scientist's choice for healing, she admits to some complexity. She notes that Christian Scientists do not themselves view their choice for treatment as a risk with a preset chance for success; rather, they view their choice as the need to assess their own ability to achieve a certain mental state that, when achieved, will *always* result in healing. "The devout Scientist believes that the risk of death from disease correctly understood and adequately prayed for is nil. But what the Scientist, devout or otherwise, is not encouraged to assess in making risk-taking choices is how likely it is that he or she will correctly understand and adequately pray for release from the condition."[2] Battin claims that even when the Christian Scientist's choice is viewed in this very different way, the church fails to provide evidence (anecdotal or otherwise) that would help a Scientist assess whether he or she can achieve the correct mental state.

Battin also admits that the ends desired by a Christian Scientist may be more than just a cure for a particular disease. She acknowledges that when a Christian Scientist has as a higher priority the goal of increasing spiritual understanding when seeking spiritual means for healing, the pursuit of this more central goal results in there being a different type of health-related choice than merely choosing between alternative methods for curing disease, and that the type of information needed in order to make this choice would also be different:

> If a believer approaches a Christian Science practitioner not to get well but in order to deepen his or her faith—as many devout Christian Scientists clearly do—then *it is not so clear that these constraints apply* [my emphasis]. Many Christian Scientists conceive of healing not as an alternative medical system at all but as a process of prayer that is part of the effort to achieve a certain spiritual condition of which a side effect, though not the central purpose, may be the restoration of health.[3]

But even after noting that many Christian Scientists do have goals other than merely curing a diseased condition, Battin argues that "by the very fact that it [the Christian Science Church] distributes testimonials that recount favorable recoveries using Christian Science healing" and "by asking Blue Cross to cover the services it renders" that "Christian Science announces and promotes itself as an alternative healing system."[4] Here she seems to be arguing that although a devout Christian Scientist does not view a health-related choice as a choice simply between alternative methods for curing disease and thus may not view base-rate information on alternative cures as relevant to this choice, *some people* would view Christian Science simply as an alternative healing method (as a result of the way Christian Science promotes itself) and would need success-rate statistics in order to decide whether to use this method.

In summary, Battin has three main criticisms of the Christian Science Church (with an emphasis on the first):

1. The Christian Scientist's health-related choice should be viewed as resembling any choice with quantifiable external likelihood of success; therefore, the church is at fault for failing to supply the success-rate information needed to make that choice.
2. Even if the Christian Scientist's choice is viewed as the need for an individual to assess his own ability to successfully carry out a healing method that *always* works when correctly executed, the church is ethically remiss for failing to inform adherents of the conditions that must obtain in a successful attempt.
3. Even though devout Christian Scientists do not view a health-related choice as a choice simply between alternative methods for curing disease, nondevout Christian Scientists and non-Christian Scientists *are* encouraged by the church to view Christian Science as an alternative healing method. Thus the church should, but does not, supply a healing-success record for outsiders to rationally assess this alternative for healing particular ailments.

In showing what is wrong with Battin's views, I first explore the nature of the choices Christian Scientists actually make and then determine the information most needed as a basis for making these choices. I show that base-rate information is irrelevant to a Christian Scientist's decision-making process and that anecdotal accounts of Christian Science healings published by the church play an important and ethically-responsible role in both the Scientist's and the non-Scientist's decision-making process. Finally, I argue that the choice of both Christian Scientists and non-Christian Scientists is not one of simply deciding between alternative approaches to curing disease but is one of deciding between alternative worldviews. The choice to adhere to a Christian Science worldview is as rationally defensible as the choice to adhere to the worldview held by medical scientists.

The Goals of a Christian Scientist

In order to determine if a Christian Scientist can and does make rational choices, it is essential to know the ends being pursued by a Christian Scientist. Once the ends are clear, it can be determined if the chosen means to reach those ends are rational. Of course, it can always be argued that such ends are really not better than some other set of ends, but such an argument becomes one of value rather than rationality.[5] And since Battin is addressing whether Christian Scientists are supplied the information needed to make rational choices, not whether the goals of Christian Scientists are worth pursuing, I focus in this section only on defining the goals themselves and not on their value relative to others' differing goals.

Since Christian Science is first and foremost a *religion* built on the teachings and life of Jesus, a Christian Scientist's goals are religious in nature. Christian Scientists attempt to follow Jesus' example in his understanding of spiritual reality and in his demonstration of it. Christian Scientists believe that Jesus' understanding of God and of man's true spiritual nature enabled him to heal both sin and sickness and that anyone's increased understanding can bring about similar results. But the *primary goal* for a Christian Scientist is to gain a more spiritualized consciousness; all positive results from achieving this goal are "added unto" him or her. Pursuing spiritual consciousness as a priority is in direct agreement with Jesus' teaching: "Seek ye first the kingdom of God . . . and all these things shall be added unto you."[6] The supreme good in life that a Christian Scientist pursues is similar to William James's characterization of the good pursued in all religious lives: "Were one asked to characterize the life of religion in the broadest and most general terms possible, one might say that it consists in the belief that there is an unseen order, and that our supreme good lies in harmoniously adjusting ourselves thereto."[7] Christian Scientists would certainly agree that their "supreme good" comes from "harmoniously adjusting" to an ordered, harmonious spiritual reality—from understanding and living a life that better reflects the qualities of a God that is defined as "Mind, Spirit, Soul, Principle, Life, Truth, Love."[8] Christian Scientists also expect and experience such materially tangible good results as physical healings after successfully adjusting to spiritual reality and becoming conscious of it. Mary Baker Eddy, the founder of the Christian Science Church, writes in the textbook studied daily by practicing Christian Scientists, "Become conscious for a single moment that Life and intelligence are purely spiritual—neither in nor of matter—and the body will then utter no complaints."[9]

Christian Scientists certainly expect healthy bodies, but only in the sense that healing material conditions is a way to demonstrate the goodness and power of God. In his recently published book, Richard Nenneman, a former editor in chief of *The Christian Science Monitor,* explains the goals of a Christian Scientist as they relate to "healthy bodies":

> For what does one pray? We have said that prayer is primarily not one of petition. If one is praying to see more of God's kingdom on earth, the prayer will usually be specific. But the demonstration the Christian Scientist is making is not one defined by the limits of the material senses—a healthy body, a better job, a bigger house, a kinder husband, or a more generous employer. These may be the things we think we need. On examination, however, a sincere Christian is forced to admit that what he or she really needs, and the only thing he or she needs, is a fuller consciousness of God's presence and power.[10]

Although a Christian Scientist may originally be motivated to pray because of an inharmonious physical or mental condition, the Christian Scientist is taught to reexamine his or her desires and to desire first and foremost additional spiritual insight, since such insight produces a much deeper and more lasting sense of well-being—a sense of well-being not contingent on particular material conditions.

Since Battin argues that the Christian Science Church "announces and promotes itself as an alternative healing system" by publishing positive accounts of healing, it is important to point out here that Christian Scientists are *directly* told that Christian Science is not to be viewed in this way, both by Mary Baker Eddy in her textbook and by authors published in the Christian Science periodicals—the very periodicals containing accounts of healing. Mary Baker Eddy writes that "the mission of Christian Science now, as in the time of its earlier demonstration, is not primarily one of physical healing. Now, as then, signs and wonders are wrought in the metaphysical healing of physical disease; but these signs are only to demonstrate its divine origin."[11]

An article published in the *Christian Science Journal* describes the healing of a blood condition using Christian Science, and the author of the article goes on to state that

> as grateful as Christian Scientists are for such healings, they don't regard spiritual healing simply as an alternative to medical or other forms of treatment. Healing is seen both as worship—a substantial way to glorify God—and as scientific proof that reality is wholly spiritual and good. Put another way, each healing of a disease, an injustice, or a sinful habit is seen as a yielding of the mistaken belief that everything is merely matter, to the reality of Spirit as the primal and only substance and cause.[12]

Christian Science does *not* simply "announce and promote itself as an alternative healing system." Rather, it views healings as a demonstration that reality is spiritual and as an important by-product of an increased understanding of this spiritual reality. If Christian Scientists' primary goal is increased spiritual understanding and if they view physical healing as a secondary benefit resulting from such increased understanding, then choosing means that result in the curing of physical conditions but fail to increase their understanding of or demonstration of spiritual reality could not be considered rational.

Base-Rate Information in a Christian Scientist's Life

Clearly, if the end pursued by a Christian Scientist is a more spiritualized consciousness, then physical healing success-rate information is of little value in the pursuit of that end. For example, an individual pursuing an advanced understanding of calculus would hardly need to know how many before her attempted such an understanding and failed to achieve it. But even assuming that such information were available, it is relevant to that individual's decision-making processes only to the degree that it points to an impossibility (or extreme unlikelihood) of that individual's achieving the desired understanding. *If* such understanding is her goal, she has no other choice but to attempt to learn calculus. No one else can learn it for her. A medical patient relies on someone other than himself to cure his illness and thus has a number of alternative experts and material methods from which to choose (each with an accompanying success-rate external to the patient). But the Christian Scientist must take responsibility for advancing his own mental state. A Christian Scientist believes that such advancing can only occur through his own study, prayers, and acts or through the help of a Christian Science practitioner's prayers.[13] Just as a student can only advance in calculus through study and practice, so a Christian Scientist can only advance through study, prayer, and practice. A Christian Scientist is certainly able to explore alternative religions or philosophies in a quest for increased spiritual consciousness, but it would not be rational to pursue medical means for such a quest, since medical practitioners make no claim to spiritual expertise.

This does not mean that Christian Scientists martyr themselves in pursuit of spiritual healing. They do expect that when they have reached a better understanding of spiritual reality, they will also be healed. There is no doubt that there are those Christian Scientists who in especially alarming situations may question their ability to achieve the spiritual growth necessary for healing. And there are also those who may not wish to dedicate themselves to what they perceive to be too much spiritual effort necessary for healing a condition known to be easily cured by medical means. But in neither of these cases would base-rate information on the success rate of a

Christian Science approach to healing make the decision to pursue medical means any easier or more informed.

In this section, I have argued against Battin's assertion that an ailing Christian Scientist faces a choice that "resembles in structure any other prudential calculation under risk" in which "various possible outcomes . . . are foreseen under specific valuations and under more or less quantifiable expectations about the likelihood of their occurrence."[14] As Battin herself points out in a later section of her chapter, Christian Scientists do *not* view themselves as making choices for which specific success rates external to themselves are relevant. Rather, they choose to live a religious way of life with spiritual growth as a goal and with physical healings as one additional benefit from gaining an increased understanding of spiritual reality.

The Role of Healing in Christian Science

Christian Scientists share and publish anecdotes of healing as a way to worship and praise God and as a way to show that a Christlike understanding of spiritual reality is being and can be demonstrated via physical healings. It is important to note that accounts of healing are never presented in isolation. They follow theological articles in the periodicals, just as such healing accounts included in the final chapter of *Science and Health* follow seventeen chapters of exposition of Christian Science. Healings are clearly viewed as the fruitage of increased spiritual understanding and as proof that Christian Science, when properly understood and applied, brings about tangible and often dramatic positive results.

The healing accounts themselves are instructive and often contain details of the Christian Scientist's experience of healing—details of what thoughts and actions resulted in a changed physical condition. The writers of such testimonials often begin their accounts with descriptions of failed approaches at healing the particular condition. They then describe the approach that finally results in healing. Sometimes failed approaches include attempted medical means and sometimes failed approaches include Christian Science study that fails to result in the mental state needed for the physical condition to be healed.

There is no doubt that such failed approaches are only included as part of what led up to an eventual healing using Christian Science and that such accounts are published within and as part of the belief system of Christian Science. But there is also no doubt that the writers are Christian Scientists and wish to encourage others to pursue Christian Science or remain committed to using it. The writers are convinced that Christian Science brings about physical healing as a side effect of advanced spiritual consciousness. Over and over, such writers follow their account of physical healing with such comments as, "While I fully appreciate the release from my physical troubles, this pales in significance in comparison with the spiritual uplifting Christian Science has brought me." Or "all of this [a child cured of a medically diagnosed terminal illness] is, however, nothing to compare with the spiritual uplifting which I have received, and I have everything to be thankful for."[15] Many testifiers stress that only when they gave up seeking mere physical relief in favor of advancing their spiritual understanding did a physical healing result and that in the end the spiritual advancement was much more valuable to them than the physical healing. It is also significant that many healing accounts are of nonphysical conditions such as loneliness, suicidal tendencies, or relationship problems.

Christian Scientists choose to share such accounts and choose to listen to and read such accounts within the context of a religious community—a community in which individual members commit to worshiping together and to helping each other better understand and demonstrate their jointly held religious beliefs. Sharing accounts of healing is a way to encourage others to use Christian Science as a means to *both* spiritual advancement and physical healing. Accounts of healing are often instructive regarding actions and mental states that brought about the healing and often describe unsuccessful approaches that preceded the eventual healing. Thus, in direct contrast to Battin, I argue that published accounts of healing are not presented by an "ethically remiss" institution simply as evidence that Christian Science is more effective at healing physical conditions than a medical approach to healing. Rather, such accounts are shared among members of the Christian Science community as part of their worship, as encouragement to others, and as instruction on how the study and practice of Christian Science can bring about both a greater (and valuable in itself) understanding of spiritual reality and an improved (but secondary) physical health.

Christian Scientists are faced daily with media accounts of disease and with a dominant medical paradigm claiming that certain diseases will cause death if not treated medically (or in many cases will cause death even with medical treatment). It is challenging, to say the least, for a practicing Christian Scientist not to catch society's fear and concern. Shared accounts of successful healing using Christian Science are one way to assure others that discouragement, apathy, or fear can and should be overcome and to help others gain a stronger sense of hope and expectation in the healing efficacy of a more spiritual way of life—a way of life that according to Christian

Scientists (and many medical professionals) results in physical healings that cannot be explained by medical scientists using a primarily materialistic theory of disease.

Battin contends that the Christian Science Church presents itself as offering an alternative health care system. In one sense, she is right, but only when health is viewed as exemplified in *both* one's spiritual and one's physical state. The Christian Science "alternative" is a religious alternative in which the spiritual and physical condition of a patient are inexorably linked. In this view, the patient's mental condition is of primary importance and plays a causal role in that patient's physical well-being. In other words, the Christian Scientist's view of "health" and "healing" is *much broader* than the secular medical view that health equates to physical well-being and that causes of disease equate primarily to biological causes.

Battin acknowledges that Christian Scientists view both the causes and the nature of disease very differently but also argues at one point that Christian Scientists accept and the church promotes "a variety of external similarities" that reinforce the claim that the Christian Science Church functions as an alternative to medical institutions. She lists the following similarities: Christian Scientists call practitioners when they have "discomforting symptoms," practitioners are listed in the Yellow Pages, appointments are made with practitioners, practitioners are paid at rates similar to physician's rates, and "Blue Cross will pay the bill."[16] I have two points to make here: First, as I have already shown, Christian Scientists themselves do not view these external similarities as reasons to view the church as an alternative to medicine. Rather, the content of what they read in both *Science and Health* and published accounts of healing directly tell them *not* to view Christian Science in this way. Second, although some Christian Science institutional practices can be viewed as externally similar to medical institutional practices, many more of its institutional practices are quite clearly dissimilar. When *all* Christian Science institutional practices are taken into account, it is quite obvious that the institutions to which the Christian Science Church presents itself as an alternative are other *church* institutions. Christian Science church buildings, published periodicals, and institutional advertisements in the Yellow Pages all present the Christian Science Church as a church—a religious institution. On Sunday morning, neither a Christian Scientist nor anyone else would view the choice to be made as one of driving to either a hospital or a Christian Science Church. And when a Christian Scientist is experiencing "discomforting symptoms," she does not at that point choose between a medical institution and the Christian Science Church. Rather, she has *already chosen* her religious alternative—she has already chosen her worldview, way of life, and the religious institution designed to promote that way of life.

Differing Worldviews

Many, including Battin, would agree that Christian Scientists do indeed make *subjectively* rational decisions. Within the context of a Christian Scientist's beliefs and goals, choosing Christian Science as a means to achieving advanced spiritual understanding, as well as the physical healing that accompanies this understanding, can be viewed as rational. But many question the objective rationality of the belief system of Christian Science itself. Is it rational to think that there is, in fact, a spiritual reality? If there is such a reality, is it rational to think that we can know or experience this reality to any degree? And even if a few individuals such as Jesus (or other high-visibility religious figures) were able to glimpse and to demonstrate the healing effect of an understanding of this spiritual reality, is it rational to expect just anyone to be able to understand and demonstrate this reality? Such questions and their possible answers go well beyond the scope of either Battin's or my project, but I do wish to address them, if only briefly, because a skeptical reader would most certainly have such questions. Battin herself, although claiming not to be challenging the verity of Christian Science beliefs, clearly writes from the perspective that a Christian Scientist's choices are at best subjectively rational but certainly not objectively rational. The rationality of the Christian Scientist's belief system is also relevant to Battin's and my project when the choice a Christian Scientist must make when deciding whether to turn to medical care is viewed as a choice between two very different sets of premises about the nature of the world and more specifically about the relationship between disease and certain mental states.

Although space does not permit me to address fully the issues and debate that surround making a choice between two very different belief systems or theories, I wish to highlight how such a choice can be viewed as being ultimately a matter of individual conscience rather than objective rationality.

Christian Scientists and medical practitioners can be viewed as practicing within two different belief systems—as adhering to two very different theories about the nature of the world and as holding very different premises about the cause of and cure for physical conditions. Practices built out of these two theories both appear to produce healing results, although as has been emphasized throughout this paper, the practice of Christian

Science also produces what Christian Scientists term advanced spiritual understanding. Christian Scientists experience healing results for themselves, observe healings in family members, and learn of others' healing experiences at Wednesday services and through Christian Science periodicals. Even Battin acknowledges that it cannot be assumed that "Christian Science healing is in fact less effective than conventional medical therapy."[17] Thus it can be argued that Christian Scientists and medical practitioners hold to two very different and conflicting sets of premises, *each of which* when practiced appears to bring about results.

Several philosophers have noted that certain practices based on ideologies that conflict with Western medical science do in fact bring about cures that cannot be explained within the medical paradigm. Paul Feyerabend, in his writings on the need for society to defend itself against science, points out that arguing that medical science "deserves a special position because it has produced results . . . is an argument only if it can be taken for granted that nothing else has ever produced results." He continues by asserting that effective methods of medical diagnosis and therapy do exist outside of the ideology of Western science.[18] William James also comments on the healing results achieved outside of science in *Varieties of Religious Experience*. In a chapter devoted to "healthy-minded" religions James lumps Christian Science in with other "mind-cures," noting that "religion in the shape of mind-cure . . . prevents certain forms of disease as well as science does, or even better in a certain class of persons.[19] And Michael Polanyi, in his writings on faith and science, has noted that "Christian Science succeeds in contesting effectively even today the interpretation of disease and healing by science."[20]

Even though Christian Scientists have accumulated a large body of well-documented evidence for healing results, the evidence for the truth of Christian Science as a theory comes both from such materially tangible healing evidence *and* from religious experience. Evidence for the existence of spiritual reality and even for mental causes of diseased physical conditions is by its very nature different from evidence used to verify physical theories within the physical sciences. In describing the reality sensed as a result of religious experience, William James writes, "It is as if there were in the human consciousness a sense of reality, a feeling of objective presence, a perception of what we may call 'something there,' more deep and more general than any of the special and particular 'senses' by which the current psychology supposes existent realities to be originally revealed."[21]

Although Christian Science and medical science are based on significantly different theories, there is *some* evidence that can be shared and discussed between those adhering to these different theories. This evidence would include the already existing documentation of physical cures achieved by those adhering to the Christian Science worldview. Evidence for these medically unexplainable cures can be found not only in anecdotal accounts but in before-and-after X rays and in documented before-and-after medical examinations. I do think a discussion between those holding to medical theories and those holding to the Christian Science worldview would be useful and beneficial to both groups, but Christian Scientists run into several potential difficulties in such a discussion. If they present evidence for physical cures to medical institutions and thus stress this evidence, they can easily be viewed as presenting themselves as a mere alternative to secular medicine. And just as importantly, such a discussion would be asymmetrical. The political, economic, and epistemic power lies with medical science institutions and not with a marginalized religious institution.

In attempting to determine the types of acceptable evidence for medically unexplainable cures or for Christian Science as a theory, secular medical scientists understandably wish to "set the rules" on what counts as valid evidence. Those within the Western science paradigm argue that evidence is most convincing when it is produced within controlled experiments and observed by skeptical onlookers. But Christian Scientists would argue that the achievement of certain mental and spiritual states cannot be "objectively" controlled and observed in the same way that physical scientists control and observe physical phenomena. As a result, evidence for Christian Scientists comes much more from their own individual experiences and from accounts by those whose lives they trust and respect. As already pointed out, both physical-healing evidence *and* religious-experience evidence go into their choosing a paradigm so different from medical science.

Once Christian Science and medical science are viewed as being two very different theories with differing premises and differing types of evidence that count as verification for these theories, the possibility of *rationally* choosing between these two theories becomes remote. As Thomas Kuhn points out, there are "significant limits to what the proponents of different theories can communicate to one another," and "the same limits make it difficult or, more likely, impossible for an individual to hold both theories in mind together and compare them point by point with each other and with nature."[22]

The inability to hold two very different theories in mind together not only results in a difficulty in choosing between the two theories but also points to why Christian Scientists do not attempt to "mix" medical and Christian Science means when faced with a health-related choice. Christian Scientists who have chosen to address their health-related concerns using the Christian Science worldview put themselves at epistemic risk when they turn to medical institutions and thus attempt to mix Christian Science premises and views with very different medical premises and views.

In the end, the main choice a Christian Scientist must make (and then commit to) is one between two differing worldviews. Deciding between two theories (each with its own internal consistency, empirical verification, and demonstrated beneficial results) becomes a matter of individual responsibility or conscience. Christian Scientists can be viewed as participating in what Polanyi terms "a community of consciences jointly rooted in the same ideals recognized by all" in which "the community becomes an embodiment of these ideals and a living demonstration of their reality."[23] As members of this community decide whether to remain within this embodiment of ideals, they decide based less on pure rationality than on what they perceive to be the value of the qualities and reality lived by other members of this community. They must depend on what general impression of rationality and spiritual worth others within this community exhibit. I argue that choosing between the belief system of Christian Scientists and that of medical scientists can only be accomplished using such *impressions* of rationality and *judgments* of spiritual worth so described by Polanyi.

Conclusion

A Christian Scientist makes health-related choices that may appear irrational to those who adhere to the worldview held by medical scientists. But when the goals of Christian Scientists are carefully examined, their "irrational" choices are easily seen as rational choices for means to achieving their goals. And when it is acknowledged that Christian Scientists offer positive accounts of healing to those who share their goals as part of religious worship and as encouragement and instruction for others in the achievement of shared goals, it can easily be argued that such positive accounts form neither an inadequate nor an unethical basis for rational choice. The choice that the Christian Scientist must make is a choice to live either by the values and worldview held within the Christian Science community or by the values and worldview held within the dominant medically oriented community. The making of this choice is a matter primarily of conscience.

Notes

1. Margaret P. Battin, *Ethics in the Sanctuary: Examining the Practices of Organized Religion* (New Haven: Yale University Press, 1990), 80.

2. Ibid., 99.

3. Ibid., 122.

4. Ibid.

5. Some moral theorists claim that questions of value *can* be answered using rationality. However, this is not the focus of either Battin's arguments or my own.

6. Matthew 6:33; Luke 12:31.

7. William James, *The Varieties of Religious Experience* (New York: Penguin, 1902), 53.

8. Mary Baker Eddy, *Science and Health with Key to the Scriptures* (Boston: The First Church of Christ, Scientist, 1906), 465.

9. Eddy, *Science and Health*, 14.

10. Richard A. Nenneman, *The New Birth of Christianity: Why Religion Persists in a Scientific Age* (San Francisco: HarperCollins, 1992), 155–156.

11. Eddy, *Science and Health*, 150.

12. Margaret Rogers, "Materialism Yielding to Spirituality," *The Christian Science Journal* 110, no. 6 (June 1992): 35.

13. When a Christian Scientist asks a Christian Science practitioner for help in achieving a more spiritualized consciousness, the practitioner prays for the Christian Scientist with the expectation that her prayers will result in the caller's experiencing a heightened sense of God's presence. Nevertheless, the caller is expected to be pursuing increased spiritual understanding himself (unless he is unable to do so).

14. Battin, *Ethics in the Sanctuary*, 80.

15. The two quotations cited are found in separate accounts of healing included in the final chapter of *Science and Health*, 610, 614.

16. Battin, *Ethics in the Sanctuary*, 120.

17. Ibid., 97. Battin quotes from a report produced by the Christian Science Church containing an empirical analysis of medical evidence in published Christian Science accounts of healing from 1969 to 1988. The authors of this report assert that over 10,000 physical healings were published in this period and that 2,337 were of medically diagnosed conditions. For more detail of the types of conditions reported as healed and of the ways in which such healing accounts are verified, see "An Empirical Analysis of Medical Evidence in Christian Science Testimonies of Healing, 1969–1988" (available upon request from the Committee on Publication, The First Church of Christ, Scientist, Boston, Massachusetts).

18. Paul Feyerabend, "How to Defend Society against Science," *Radical Philosophy* 11 (1975): 6.

19. James, *Varieties of Religious Experience*, 122. James also wrote a letter to the *Boston Transcript* in March 1894 defending the right of the Christian Scientist or any other mind curer to practice healing: *I assuredly hold no brief for any of these healers, and must confess that my intellect has been unable to assimilate their theories, so far as I have heard them given. But their facts are patent and startling; and*

anything that interferes with the multiplication of such facts, and with our freest opportunity of observing and studying them, will, I believe, be a public calamity.

20. Michael Polanyi, *Science, Faith, and Society* (1946; Chicago: University of Chicago Press, 1964), 66.

21. James, *Varieties of Religious Experience,* 58.

22. Thomas Kuhn, "Objectivity, Value Judgment, and Theory Choice," in *The Essential Tension* (Chicago: University of Chicago Press, 1977), 338.

23. Polanyi, *Science, Faith, and Society,* 56.

3

Put Up or Shut Up?

Countering the Defense of Christian Science

Margaret P. Battin

Christian Science, I've argued, raises compelling moral issues about the ways in which religious groups treat their members. To be sure, Christian Science is hardly alone in this respect—many religious groups raise troubling issues of this sort—but Christian Science presses the issue of "informed consent" in accepting and refusing medical treatment in a particularly acute way. I see this as a troubling ethical dilemma.

Peggy DesAutels, in her important, spirited reply to my charge, argues that this is not the problem I think it is. She claims that the worldviews of the Christian Scientist and the non-Scientist are at odds. One is "matter based," as it might be put, the other "spirit based." Thus, she argues, we cannot impose ordinary ethical expectations of informed consent on the church, on its practitioners, or on its believing members who seek help in easing or curing their illnesses by turning to Christian Science prayer.

I think DesAutels's argument fails. It fails because Christian Science still seems to want to have it both ways—to function both as a system of alternative medical treatment and, at the same time, as a religious system rooted in distinctive metaphysical beliefs about the nature of body and mind; this is the dual "pitch" made to long-term members and prospective converts alike.[1] But DesAutels's argument is so sensitive to the beliefs of practicing Christian Scientists that I'd like to try to draw out the consequences of what she says as a way of showing what the real dilemma is, as I see it, for Christian Science in the contemporary world. DesAutels undercuts her own argument, I believe, by treating it as the end of the conversation. Having argued that Scientists and non-Scientists are operating from two different worldviews, she takes that to be the end of the matter; but I think that she instead introduces new, larger issues. Thus her remarks should be treated as the beginning of a further conversation, to be pursued here, not as the end of the current one.

Let me get right to the point. My challenge to Christian Science was, in essence, a "put-up-or-shut-up" one—either prove that Christian Science healing is effective or stop making the claim that it *is* effective and, furthermore, stop employing practical strategies (e.g., charging fees for healing and having Blue Cross pay the bill[2]) that suggest that it is effective. The ethical challenge posed to Christian Science requires that it face a practical dilemma that looks like this:

Christian Science must either

1. prove the effectiveness of Christian Science healing
2. or abandon all self-presentation that Christian Science healing is effective.

Not to do one or the other of these, I have argued, is a violation of what would in other areas be called professional responsibility and would in particular violate canons of informed consent. It is morally wrong to encourage people—either current church members or prospective converts—to use Christian Science healing in preference to conventional medicine to cure their ills if you cannot provide them with adequate information, specifically including information about the rates of effectiveness of the two forms of treatment, for making such a choice. It is wrong, in other words, to claim that prayer is a "more dependable form of healing"[3] if you cannot actually establish that this is the case. The church does attempt to present its views (for example by preparing videos for paramedics or other medical personnel who might come in contact with Christian Scientists), but this is a long way from providing testable, scientifically confirmable results.

DesAutels has argued that Christian Science does not face such a dilemma, since the objective of Christian Science practice is not primarily to cure disease but rather to attain a state of spiritualized consciousness from which healing then naturally flows. Indeed, to the believing Scientist this does not seem to be a dilemma at all, since the Scientist believes that attainment of this altered state of consciousness results in physical healing, indeed, *always* results in healing if this more spiritualized consciousness is really attained. But Christian Science cannot have it both ways: It cannot claim to be a religious system and, at the same time, base its appeal on claims that it is effective in curing disease.[4] This leaves us with the dilemma set out above. Thus I would like to explore what Christian Science faces in pursuing one alternative or the other—to explore the routes DesAutels claims cannot and need not be taken. I see such exploration as the only way of preserving the church's moral integrity in the face of objections that it violates the basic canon of informed consent, a canon as essential in religious practice, I have argued, as in other areas of professional ethics. To look at these options is thus to pursue the conversation DesAutels incorrectly thought would come to an end with the assertion that Scientists and non-Scientists simply have different worldviews. They may in fact have different worldviews, but this is hardly the end of the story.

Two options are open to Christian Science. The first is to prove the medical claims. Suppose Christian Science elected to try to *prove* that its healing practices are effective. Doing so would necessarily involve comparative empirical studies of outcomes of Christian Science healing versus available alternatives. This is not to try to combine or blend medicine and healing, as would indeed be problematic if, as DesAutels claims, different worldviews are involved, but to look at the outcomes of each independent form of treatment.

Conducting comparative empirical studies would clearly constitute a different way of establishing efficacy than the ways now recognized by the church, which are limited to direct personal experience of one's own healings and first-person accounts by others. Christian Science could not continue to rely on its practice of giving testimonials, on its weighty record, *A Century of Christian Science Healing,*[5] or even on its own so-called empirical study, an ample collection and analysis of anecdotal reports of cases of healing between 1969 and 1988,[6] since such stories and accounts cannot establish base rates of illness and cure or provide any reliable comparative data. In particular, they cannot establish the sometimes tacit, sometimes explicit assumption that Christian Science healing is effective where conventional medicine is not, especially in the most serious cases, even though many Scientists have what they describe as extremely powerful, convincing experiences of such healings, sometimes occurring in cases in which there has been antecedent diagnosis and failed medical treatment.

What would be required to try to *prove* Christian Science's claims are rigorously designed studies comparing rates of illness and cure for those using Christian Science prayer, conventional medical treatment, and no treatment, and, perhaps, nonconventional or countercultural forms of medical treatment as well. Such studies can be either general—comparing, for example, lost work days, disability, or death rates for matched samples from each group—or specific, comparing outcomes by identified condition, including, say, influenza, diabetes, breast cancer, hepatitis, or myocardial infarction. Comparative empirical studies of Christian Science treatment have been proposed in the past, including, for example, by Dr. Isabelle V. Kendig, then chief clinical psychologist at the National Institute of Mental Health, who in 1957 sought to compare the health records of a group of one hundred Christian Scientist inductees in the U.S. Navy with matched non-Scientist controls. (The study was blocked, according to Robert Peel, not by the church, which said it had no objection to the project, but by the government, apparently leery [in Kendig's words] of anything having to do with religion.[7]) But the church has opposed or failed to support most calls for rigorous comparative studies, usually arguing that randomization would not be possible, that treatment by prayer and by conventional medical procedure could not be offered in double-blind fashion, and that it would be destructive to the spirituality of believing Scientists to subject them to conventional medical diagnosis, even if they were not to be treated.

Nevertheless, one route open to the church is to work with conventional medical practitioners in designing studies that as far as possible overcome these obstacles and provide objective results about outcomes, both in general and on a condition-by-condition basis. This might require some ingenuity in study design; for example, comparisons could be based on symptom clusters rather than diagnosed conditions; or both Scientist and non-Scientist volunteers could be solicited to undergo diagnosis but not be informed of the results; or large populations could be followed under careful matching for all health-risk factors; and so on.[8] Furthermore, it would require some sensitivity to conceptual issues, for example, in stipulating what counts as morbidity, health, dysfunction, remission, and cure; and so on. Non-Scientists as well as Scientists might have to rethink their conceptions of medical benefit, risk, and outcome. Designing such studies may be less difficult for minor conditions than for major, life-threatening illnesses, or more difficult in conditio· s that include psychiatric as well as physical illness. Nevertheless, I think it is possible to construct at least some informative, suggestive studies, at least if there is adequate cooperation between Scientists and non-Scientists in their design.

The second option that is open to Christian Science is to augment the religious claims and abandon claims to effectiveness. The alternative route for Christian Science would be to reinforce its identity as a *religion*, dropping practices (e.g., charging fees for healing and having Blue Cross pay the bill) that suggest it is essentially an alternative medical system. (Much of what DesAutels says suggests that it should be understood primarily in this way, that is, as a religion rather than as an alternative medical system.) Doing so would be no easier than designing adequate controlled trials, since dropping these self-presentation features would involve departing from much of Christian Science's history and current practice. Among other things, this would mean dropping the practice of having testimonials about healing serve as a major part of Wednesday worship services, discontinuing the practice of printing testimonials of healings in church publications, and, of course, dropping reimbursement by Blue Cross. Worship services would focus on the achievement of enlightened consciousness, and the publication of testimonials by Scientists would serve to show how they came to achieve such consciousness. Prayer practices would not be initiated for the purpose of healing. Furthermore, prayer would not be primarily initiated in conditions of illness but would be engaged in for its own intrinsic value, without reference to its side effects in healing. Turning to prayer would no longer be the normal, institutionally supported response *in time of illness;* instead, prayer would simply be encouraged all the time (as it already is) but not redoubled or specialized for times of illness. Nor would the group maintain any further practice (though it is often insisted that this is not the case) of prohibiting or discouraging members from turning to conventional medicine in time of illness. In these ways, Christian Science would be transformed into a religious group more like, say, Buddhism in character, in which the central objective of practice is the attainment and maintenance of a nonmaterialist, spiritualist worldview. If Scientists also wished to believe that this spiritualized consciousness also results in physical healing, that would be their business; but the church would no longer encourage prayer or the quest for more spiritualized consciousness *in order to be healed,* either as a primary or a secondary effect.

Neither course of action would seem to preserve much of what we now think of as Christian Science; they may seem to be extreme and unrealistic. Furthermore, DesAutels has already offered objections to both of them: against the first, that the effectiveness of Christian Science healing is not open to empirical proof; and against the second, that Christian Science's self-presentation does not delude either current members or prospective ones, since its dedication to the achievement of a more spiritualized understanding is explicit or presupposed in all its presentations and practices, and healing is already understood by all as a by-product or secondary goal. But DesAutels's objections are both open to counterargument. To the first, it would be possible, though not perhaps easy, to actually test the efficacy of Christian Science healing practices in an unbiased way. To the second, Christian Science's current self-presentation can delude both current members and prospective future ones. This is true whether or not their "worldviews" are different or similar to those of non-Scientists, that is, whether they do or do not have materialist outlooks. Rather, what counts here are the outcomes of the practices in question and their effects on people who engage in them, including long-term members, new members who convert in order to cure illness that medical science has been unable to treat, and, where decisions to pursue Christian Science healing rather than medical care have been made on their behalf, children. That leaves Christian Science facing the dilemma outlined above—either put up or shut up. Either *prove* that healing is effective (and not just by adding up anecdotal stories) or stop claiming that it is. Though these two positions may seem to be extreme ones, they are the only two ways to resolve the moral dilemma Christian Science now faces.

But this seems to suggest that the two routes, (1) to put up by proving that healing is effective or (2) to shut up by dropping claims that it is, are equally defensible as courses of action for the church. However, I do not think this is the case; in order to understand this, is it necessary to look at the relationship between the two.

Consider what might happen if the church pursued the first course of action: It would decide to "put up" by providing evidence and so would be willing to cooperate in the design and execution of the comparative studies described above. These would be three-armed trials of Christian Science healing versus conventional medical treatment versus nontreatment, including both general studies of outcomes across populations and targeted studies of specific conditions, and might even include additional arms for various nonconventional medical therapies. I harbor no illusions that it would be easy to construct a fully rigorous study acceptable to both Scientists and practitioners of conventional medicine, even with maximal good will and genuine commitment to open exploration on both sides, but I do think it would be possible for such a study or groups of studies to produce quite suggestive results.

But now consider what the results might be: There are three principal possibilities. First, comparative studies might show that Christian Science appears to offer no benefits, either in general or for specific conditions, over conventional medical treatment or nontreatment: Christian Scientists have more symptoms, more illnesses, more sustained illnesses, and they die sooner. Second, such studies might instead show that Christian Science produces better results than standard medical treatment, both in general or for specific groups of conditions: Christian Scientists have fewer symptoms, fewer illnesses, shorter illnesses, and live longer. Third, the results might show that Christian Science offers benefit over nontreatment, but not over standard medical treatment, or benefit over standard medical treatment but not, at least in some conditions, over nontreatment, and so on. (At the moment, we have virtually no reliable data about any of these claims, except certain comparisons of outcomes of standard medical treatment and nontreatment.[9]) Nevertheless, regardless of the outcomes of these studies, Christian Science would risk little by cooperating in such studies, at least insofar as it identifies itself as a religion: Neither "good," "neutral," nor "bad" results can damage the central religious claim that the ultimate objective of religious life is to achieve a more spiritualized consciousness. This is the claim that, in DesAutels's view, should be taken as central, and it is right in concert with the assertion she quotes from Mary Baker Eddy that "the mission of Christian Science now, as in the time of its earlier demonstration, is not primarily one of physical healing." Thus far, Christian Science has little to lose; it is protected whichever way the studies turn out. Furthermore, even if the studies were to show that Scientist prayer has worse outcomes than conventional medicine or nontreatment, this would still not refute the claim that spiritualized consciousness always results in healing; it would merely undermine the claim that it is prudent to think one can attain such consciousness in an attempt to cure disease. Thus it would undercut the practice of seeking aid in prayer during times of illness in order to attain cure, though it need not discourage or preclude the practice of seeking aid in prayer not only in illness but at all times of one's life. Indeed, if the group is a *religious* group, this might seem to be a gain: Prayer would cease to be valued for extrinsic purposes and would be valued wholly for intrinsic ones. In the bargain, of course, this change would protect both loyal Christian Scientists and prospective converts from practices that would do them no good.

After all, the real test of whether Christian Science sees itself as a religious group rather than an alternative medical system is whether, as a group, it would continue to pursue spiritualized consciousness if it were demonstrated that attaining it did *not* result in healing. Thus cooperating in studies of the efficacy of Scientist prayer, as well as working to ensure that those studies were designed without bias and would yield intelligible results, would enhance Christian Science's self-understanding as well as reinforce its spiritual claims.

But suppose Christian Science, when faced with the dilemma outlined above, were instead to begin by pursuing alternative 2, to "shut up" by emphasizing only the religious claims and rejecting any attempt to prove the efficacy of Christian Science healing. It would thus retreat from all self-presentation practices that might suggest that healing is effective, like the use of testimonials, the avoidance of conventional medicine, and the use of Blue Cross to pay bills for prayer. It would of course undergo substantial changes, as remarked above, in moving away from much of its traditional and current practice, as reference to health benefits dropped out of the picture. But this would be to reinforce the centrality of prayer designed to achieve a more spiritualized consciousness. Presumably, then, Christian Scientists, no longer pursuing prayer in order to achieve health, would come to use prayer for enhanced spiritual life but would probably rely on conventional medicine in times of illness, or perhaps turn to unconventional therapies or forgo any sort of treatment altogether.

As before, several different things could happen: First, Christian Scientists' health prospects could be improved; second, Christian Scientists' health prospects could remain about the same; or third, Christian Scientists' prospects could grow worse, depending, of course, on whether Christian Science prayer has actually turned out to be effective, neutral, or damaging in comparison to conventional or nonconventional medical treatment or nontreatment for various kinds of illness. *But Christian Scientists would have no way of knowing which was the case.* It could be that the church, in choosing to "shut up," that is, to cease making claims about the efficacy of healing, had elected a course of action that would make its members and prospective converts worse off, or it could be that they were better off (or worse off for some disease conditions but better off for others), but in the absence of the comparative studies considered above, neither the church, its members, nor anybody else would have any reliable way of knowing this. (This, of course, is the current state of affairs.) But insofar as the moral injunction the church must respond to in the first place is the accusation that it violates canons of informed consent by not making or attempting to make available to its members and prospective members the kind of information that will allow them to make prudent choices about their own lives, including whether or not to turn to Christian Science prayer in time of illness, this course of action *still* runs afoul of this injunction.

Thus it is not just an open option whether the church should pursue alternative 1 or alternative 2, whether it should "put up" or "shut up." Although the church may eventually be morally obliged to shut up if it cannot put up, it ought not merely shut up without some sincere attempt to provide concrete evidence concerning the efficacy of its practices, that is, to determine whether the healing practices it now employs may not be efficacious in some or all conditions. It already tries to do this (that is what its testimonies of healings and its own "empirical study" are meant to do, provide evidence that prayer really works), but it does not try to do so in rigorously scientific ways. Yet not to try to establish the efficacy of prayer (or establish that it is not effective after all) is to shortchange not only believing members and prospective converts, but all other persons who now rely on conventional or unconventional medicine or who avoid treatment altogether.

There is another way to put this. If Christian Science knows a secret—or rather, as it believes, a "demonstrable science"—about what is conventionally labeled illness and disease, this is knowledge of paramount importance for everyone, not just Christian Scientists. After all, everyone is subject to illness and disease, and these conditions can cause immense suffering and loss in the lives of any person. Given the importance of any form of real knowledge about illness and disease, regardless of its origin, a group that had access to that knowledge would be morally obliged to explore whether its knowledge is in fact a reliable, trustworthy, genuine form of knowledge, indeed, a demonstrable "science," as it claims. To keep it as a secret for the religiously initiated would seem perverse, even if it might eventually turn out that the knowledge can be effectively used only by those who accept the background religious view. Of course, at the moment, neither Christian Scientists nor outside detractors can know whether its claims are true. To retreat before public criticism of its practices into a more insular religiosity would be the less morally defensible course, one that would make itself still more vulnerable to the initial moral objection brought against it; to try to explore the truths it believes would be the more defensible and principled one. After all, Christian Science, as I argued earlier, has little to lose (except its current indefensible ambivalence) by cooperating with medical science in exploring its claims. Even if its claims are not supported, Christian Science can still survive as a religious group with a commitment to prayer and the attainment of a nonmaterialist worldview, but it has a great deal to lose by *not* doing so.

To be sure, a comprehensive, well-designed set of studies could also have a great deal to say about the nature of self-limiting conditions, iatrogenic disease, and the placebo effect, and on these grounds alone would be of value. But it would also have a great deal to say about (religious) claims, which conventional medical science now simply ignores. Thus, in reply to DesAutels's interesting and sensitive remarks, I would encourage her not to treat the alleged difference in worldviews between Scientists and non-Scientists as a conversation stopper but to recognize that this is the beginning of a conversation that would do well for both Scientists and non-Scientists to continue.

Notes

1. See Joan C. Callahan's extensive exploration of this issue in "Christian Science Healings: An Alternative Health Care System?" *Journal of Social Philosophy* 26, no. 3 (Winter 1995): 105–111.

2. About twenty-five major insurance companies cover charges for Christian Science healing. For at least some Blue Cross plans, if Blue Cross is part of a required employee plan and the employer requires Blue Cross to provide some form of coverage for Christian Science treatment, Blue Cross will do so, but not otherwise.

3. Nathan A. Talbot, "Medicine and the Return to Christian Science," *Christian Science Sentinel* 94, no. 8 (1992): 29.

4. Callahan, "Christian Science Healings."

5. *A Century of Christian Science Healing* (Boston: The Christian Science Publishing Society, 1966).

6. Committee on Publication, "An Empirical Analysis of Medical Evidence in Christian Science Testimonies of Healing, 1969–1988," The First Church of Christ, Scientist, 175 Huntington Avenue, Boston, Mass. 02115.

7. Robert Peel, *Spiritual Healing in a Scientific Age* (San Francisco: Harper & Row, 1987), 188–189.

8. In particular, such studies would have to be designed to try to take account of Christian Science's concern that the conventional diagnosis and naming of disease tends to reinforce it, as well as the tradition's injunction against "numbering the people." "Numbering the people" was prohibited by Mary Baker Eddy in the context of measuring church growth, but it is sometimes understood to prohibit keeping statistics and other forms of data about individuals.

9. Asser and Swan's comparison of outcomes in children for whom medical treatment was not provided for religious reasons and standard survival rates (discussed in chap. 1 of this volume) is a case in point, but it involves limited and selected rather than randomized samples. Seth M. Asser and Rita Swan, "Child Fatalities from Religion-Motivated Medical Neglect," *Pediatrics* 101, no. 4 (April 1998): 624–629.

4

Putting Up

Peggy DesAutels

I am especially grateful to Margaret Battin for her willingness to engage in a sustained conversation on ethics and Christian Science. She has taken the time to research some of the actual claims, practices, and beliefs of Christian Scientists, and as a result, her concerns and criticisms are more sophisticated than most. Nonetheless, Battin remains in the grip of the medical paradigm. The type of information she maintains should be "put up" by the Christian Science Church—as a way of proving that Christian Science healing is effective—is the type of information appropriate only to the medical model of health, healing, and disease. Christian Scientists do "put up" in ways that are more than adequate for the type of choice that must be made—the choice to embrace the Christian Science worldview and resulting way of life. Christian Scientists have been writing about the quality of their lives and the healings that take place within these lives for well over a century. These narrative accounts supply the *qualitative* information most necessary for those needing to choose between a Christian Science way of life and other ways of life.

Battin accuses the Christian Science church of being ethically remiss for failing to "prove" the healing effectiveness of a Christian Science approach to healing. According to Battin, Christian Scientists should only claim healing effectiveness (and should only publish accounts of healing) after "putting up," that is, proving their claims. This proof, says Battin, would involve "rigorously designed studies comparing rates of illness and cure for those using Christian Science prayer, conventional medical treatment, and no treatment, and perhaps, nonconventional or countercultural forms of medical treatment as well." She argues that it is impossible for Christian Scientists to make rational, informed health-related decisions without comparing Christian Science cure rates to those of medical science and alternative approaches for each of the various diseases. Throughout our conversation, Battin's main point has been and continues to be that the Christian Science Church is "violating canons of informed consent" by providing only accounts of healing success. She sees two ways that the Christian Science Church can extricate itself from its moral predicament, either by proving "the effectiveness of Christian Science healing" through "rigorous comparative studies" or by abandoning "all self-presentation that Christian Science healing is effective." I will address these suggestions one at a time and will show that neither is tenable, let alone morally required.

I wish to begin by making two very general points. First, it is only rational to pursue information that is obtainable. There are any number of reasons why the "rigorous" studies advocated by Battin would be impossible to perform. Rigorous studies of a population's disease and cure rates are only statistically valid when conducted on large populations, but the Christian Science population is small. Effective comparative studies need carefully matched samples, but it is impossible to ensure that a particular population matches in relevant health-related ways to the Christian Science population.[1] (For example, do matched samples consist of nondrinking, nonsmoking churchgoers who are early-morning meditators, reasonably well-off financially, and breathing air with pollution levels found primarily in California and Massachusetts?) Perhaps most importantly, Christian Scientists consider most medical diagnoses and interventions to be detrimental to the effectiveness of a Christian Science approach, but disease by disease comparative studies must, of necessity, involve medical diagnoses. These are just a few of the more glaring problems associated with conducting the empirical studies recommended by Battin.

Second, even if some of the more "indirect" studies advocated by Battin could be conducted and at least some of the information she recommends could be obtained, decision theorists themselves have pointed out that it is not *always* rational for decision makers to seek and then evaluate more information prior to making a choice. Rather, it is rational for an agent to obtain additional information only when the benefits of seeking and evaluating the information outweigh the costs. Christian Scientists themselves do not want to know the information Battin attempts to force upon them. They have quite rationally decided that this information is not the type of information of ultimate value to them; the costs of obtaining and evaluating this particular type of information outweigh the benefits to their decision-making processes.

Before I address the kind of information that *is* relevant to a Christian Scientist's health-related choices, I wish to bring more mainstream discussions of informed consent to bear on Battin's claim that the Christian Science Church and its members do not meet "ordinary ethical expectations of informed consent." I assume that when Battin refers to "ordinary" expectations of informed consent, she refers to expectations like the ones that are found within medical settings and are described, discussed, and debated in recent court rulings and in the bioethics literature. I am surprised that she would accuse Christian Scientists of failing to meet these expectations. Why? Because so little is expected of physicians. In his discerning comments on Canterbury versus Spence, Jay Katz does not exaggerate when he notes that "the law of informed consent is substantially mythic and fairy tale-like."[2] Anyone familiar with this court ruling knows that it sanctions physicians' continuing in such practices as downplaying risks (or leaving them entirely undiscussed) whenever the physician determines that disclosure will have a deleterious effect on a patient's recovery; communicating information in such a way that patients will "consent" to the treatments the physician deems best for the patient; and omitting mention of "commonly known" risks (such as the increased risk of infection from hospital stays) even when such risks are quite significant. In summary, it is considered legally and ethically acceptable for a physician to withhold or present biased information under a wide variety of circumstances, whenever the physician deems such withholding or presenting to be of therapeutic benefit.

Nevertheless, let us imagine an informed consent "fairy tale" for a moment. Let us imagine a physician who conscientiously informs a patient not only of all the known medical alternatives and their associated risks/benefits but also of all the "commonly known" risks associated with hospital stays, anesthesia, surgery, and so on. In this tale, does the physician inform the patient of approaches to health and alternative worldviews that *conflict* with the medical paradigm? Nowhere in the bioethics literature, not even in the most fairy tale–like pieces, have I found this to be an "ethical requirement of informed consent." Informed consent practices take place within a context of shared assumptions. Just as informed consent within the context of medicine does not involve comparisons to health alternatives outside of the medical context, so informed consent within the context of Christian Science does not require comparisons to health alternatives outside of the Christian Science context. This is as it should be. Medical practitioners are experts only within a medical context and Christian Scientists are experts only within a Christian Science context. It would, in fact, be ethically *irresponsible* to claim an expertise one does not have and should not be expected to have.

The ideal of informed consent fits well with the goals of a liberal society such as ours. In theory, such morally reprehensible states of affairs as coercion, paternalism, and brainwashing can be avoided when agents are not only allowed (by governments or institutions) to make autonomous choices but are provided with the "unbiased facts" most relevant to these choices. But in spite of the well-meaning intentions of those who advocate informed consent, it is no accident that such rulings as Canterbury versus Spence back off in practice from its abstract requirements. Agents cannot choose the conditions under which they make "autonomous" choices (e.g., cultural conditions, economic realities, or power relations); they cannot avoid an inherent bias in the presentation of information (e.g., through what is selected and omitted or through how the information is worded); they cannot avoid the necessity of trusting and relying on "experts" in their day-to-day lives; and due to time constraints on all actual day-to-day "rational" decisions, they cannot avoid taking decision-making mental shortcuts.

One response, then, to Battin's accusation—that Christian Scientists are ethically remiss for failing to provide what she considers to be the "unbiased" information necessary for making rational health care decisions—is to point out how unjust it is to demand that Christian Scientists "put up" more "unbiased" information than is asked of those in medical and other "ordinary" decision-making settings. This said, however, I would like to challenge her assumption that the provision of disease cure rates results in informed and unbiased health care decision making. Information consisting solely of disease cure rates is biased toward the medical model of health care. When health and healing are viewed from a Christian Science perspective, the most appropriate information for Christian Scientists is anecdotal and qualitative.

As I pointed out in a previous chapter, Christian Scientists do not choose between Christian Science "cures" and medical "cures" on a disease-by-disease basis. Rather, Christian Scientists choose to embrace a Christian Science worldview, and the way of life (including the health-related practices) that is embedded within and arises from this worldview. A Christian Scientist can and should reflect on whether to embrace (or continue to embrace) this worldview and way of life. And one aspect of this choice can be based on the physiological health experienced in her own and other Christian Scientists' lives. At the risk of being overly repetitive, let me reiterate that the overall quality of a Christian Scientist's life is characterized by a well-being that is both physiological and spiritual.

Although religious beliefs and commitments are, ostensibly, morally "permissible" in a liberal society such as ours, most bioethicists dismiss the view that quality of life (health) is inexorably tied to spiritual advancement and thus consider choices based on this view to be irrational. But Battin goes even farther than many bioethicists by viewing health *solely* in medical terms. For medical science, health is nothing more than disease management, and measurements of health care effectiveness are nothing more than measurements of how effectively a health care system controls physiological pathologies. But healing, health, and well-being are not reducible to objective (scientific) measurements of altered pathologies. The point I am making here is no different from the position espoused by the World Health Organization (WHO)—that health should be broadly construed as consisting of physical, mental, and social well-being.

Battin's suggested focus on cure rates of various diseases fails to take mental and social well-being into account. If, for example, it turns out that Christian Scientists tend to experience higher quality lives overall than those who depend heavily on physician-prescribed drugs and medical technologies, cure rates would fail to supply this information. What are most needed are narrative accounts and qualitative studies of the lives of Christian Scientists. Christian Scientists supply the narrative accounts in their periodicals, at their Wednesday evening church meetings, and in casual and family settings. Broader, more formal qualitative studies have not been conducted but could be. Such studies could examine the degree to which Christian Scientists experience (subjectively) physical, mental, and social well-being. Results from studies such as these would indeed be "suggestive." But they would not be (nor should they be) empirical studies modeled after those found within the medical paradigm. And such quality-of-life studies are not *ethically required* for day-to-day health-related choices embedded within particular worldviews and ways of life. If they were, few actual way-of-life choices involving consequences for one's health would be rational, since most of us adhere rather unreflectively to a particular culture's assumptions and way of life.

Of course, as a philosophy professor, I am the first to advocate the "examined" life; but no institution/government is *ethically required* to provide members/citizens with alternative ways-of-life and studies that examine the relative merits of these ways of life in terms of physical, mental, and social well-being. If, in fact, reflecting on and then choosing from radically different ways of life (and radically different ways of approaching health) is not ethically required but nonetheless a "good thing to do," Christian Scientists will come out ahead of most medical patients. Christian Scientists are always well aware of the fact that they can choose the medical paradigm—that they can choose to value and avail themselves of medical studies and medical cure-rate information—and they quite consciously choose not to do so. They choose a life that emphasizes instead the physical, mental, and social health that accompanies spiritual insight, spiritual growth, and spiritual healing.

The day-to-day behaviors of committed Christian Scientists not only include prayer and church-related activities but also exclude the use of drugs, alcohol, and cigarettes. Members of the Christian Science Church commit themselves to avoiding addictive substances and addictive behaviors of all sorts. The social condition of Christian Scientists usually includes high levels of education and income. When these generally health-promoting behavioral patterns and social traits are combined with the physical, mental, and relationship-oriented *healings* that Christian Scientists report experiencing, there is ample "suggestive" evidence that the quality and type of health experienced as a result of adhering to the Christian Science worldview and way of life is high. Indeed, *rational* people could and do choose this worldview and the full range of health-related practices associated with this way of life.

I will close this reply to Battin by commenting briefly on her proposal that one ethical option for Christian Scientists is to "shut up"—to "abandon all self-presentation that Christian Science healing is effective." According to her, this would include "dropping the practice of having testimonials about healing serve as a major part of Wednesday worship services" and "discontinuing the practice of printing testimonials of healings in church publications." Battin appears to have forgotten that Christian Science church services and daily study also incorporate healing accounts from the Bible. I take it that healing accounts in the Old and New Testaments would also have to be deleted from services and study sessions. I also take it that *no* religion, Christian Science or otherwise, should incorporate the Bible's healing accounts into its services or belief system without the disclaimer that "it may be dangerous to one's health" to try such religious-based healing at home. Or perhaps Christian Scientists, Catholics, and Protestants should discontinue the practice of reading the Bible altogether?

Battin appears to be defending the view that we shouldn't tell each other instructive or inspirational stories of any sort unless we provide related "scientific" evidence for the effectiveness of the approaches taken in the stories. She also appears to be defending the view that even in religious settings, only medically defined health and healing should be discussed. But deciding the kind of health and healing most worth having and determining what counts as proof of healing effectiveness is not nor ever can be the sole purview of those who, like Battin, worship at the altar of medical materialism. Need I remind Battin that in spite of medical advancements, all human beings face death? And that prior to death, all humans must decide what most contributes to a life worth living? Health does matter to Christian Scientists, and they do expect to experience it; but what most matters to Christian Scientists are the deeply *spiritual* aspects of health and healing experienced during (and after) life here on earth.

Now it is time for me to shut up.

Notes

1. In an earlier chapter Margaret Battin refers to a study purporting to show that Christian Scientists have shorter life expectancies than non-Christian Scientists. (See William Franklin Simpson, Ph.D., "Comparative Longevity in a College Cohort of Christian Scientists," *Journal of the American Medical Association,* September 22, 1989, 1657–1658.) The study was based on alumni records from Principia College, a college for Christian Scientists, and from the University of Kansas, the "control group." This study was significantly flawed, however. First, Simpson assumed that all graduates of Principia College belonged to the Christian Science population. However, a significant number of Principia College graduates do not consider themselves to be practicing Christian Scientists. Second, Principia College stays in close contact with most of its graduates and can account for the whereabouts of most of them. The University of Kansas, on the other hand, had a significantly greater number of graduates who were unaccounted for than did Principia College. It would make sense to think that many graduates who were unaccounted for by the University of Kansas were unaccounted for *because* they had died. But for purposes of the study, "the missing students from the University of Kansas were assumed to have the same mortality rate as their same-sex classmates for whom records exist" (Simpson, 1658).

2. Jay Katz, "Physicians and Patients: A History of Silence," in *Contemporary Issues in Bioethics,* ed. Tom L. Beauchamp and LeRoy Walters, 4th ed. (Belmont, Calif.: Wadsworth, 1994), 148.

5

Challenging Medical Authority

Larry May

As a member of a hospital ethics committee in a city with a very large Christian Science population, I have seen firsthand the stalemate that exists between Christian Scientists and physicians, especially concerning the treatment of Christian Science children.[1] Physicians claim that it is a violation of their professional duties to allow those children to suffer who could be prevented from suffering by medical treatment. Christian Scientists claim that it is a violation of their religious freedom to be forced to subject their children to medical treatment in violation of their religious beliefs. The stalemate is made more tragic because neither physicians nor Christian Scientists want children to suffer or die, yet Christian Scientists refuse even to have their sick children diagnosed for fear that the physicians will try to force them to accept medical treatment. Diverging from most discussion of this topic, in this essay I consider the Christian Science refusal cases as exemplifying a conflict of groups over authority within a pluralistic society. I offer a temporary solution to this stalemate that exemplifies the notion of a communitarian-negotiated compromise.

In the first section of this essay, I present two contrasting cases of Christian Scientists who have refused medical treatment for their children. In the second section I rehearse some of the main doctrines and arguments espoused by Christian Scientists who refuse medical treatment. In the third section I attempt to explain why physicians in the United States are so strongly committed to the belief that they must be the exclusive authorities in matters of health. In the fourth section I discuss the problem of conflicts of belief in a pluralistic society, and I apply such a framework to the Christian Science refusal cases. In the final section, I suggest briefly how medical socialization should be changed so that doctors come to recognize the legitimacy of other forms of authority. And I suggest how this change,

71

when conjoined with a corresponding change in the socialization of Christian Science community members, might resolve the current stalemate on the Christian Science refusal cases.

Two Christian Science Refusal Cases

Let us consider a case that most doctors and lawyers consider a good illustration of why we should not give equal respect and treatment to the Christian Science community. On a Thursday evening in early April 1986, two-year-old Robyn Twitchell ate a normal dinner but experienced severe pain and vomiting shortly after dinner. The pain and vomiting continued into Friday and Robyn's parents, both committed Christian Scientists, consulted several church officials who determined that Robyn's pain was in his lower abdomen. On Saturday, after another day of intense pain and vomiting, Christian Science practitioner Nancy Calkins came to the Twitchell house to pray for Robyn, who was still unable to hold down food or liquids. On Monday a Christian Science nurse was called who also ministered to Robyn. By Tuesday evening Robyn Twitchell died. An autopsy was conducted and it was determined that Robyn had a bowel obstruction, which, in the opinion of one physician, "could have been readily corrected by surgery with an almost one hundred percent chance of success."[2]

The mainstream position in medicine and law is that even in a pluralistic society a line needs to be drawn at the point where respecting a religious minority culture clearly jeopardizes the well-being of children. Indeed, what makes the case of Robyn Twitchell so tragic is that a relatively simple operation could have saved his life. The fact that his parents refused even to secure a medical diagnosis meant that they were completely unaware of how seriously ill their son was. Indeed, in another highly publicized case, the parents whose failure to secure a medical diagnosis and simple treatment resulted in the death of their child have subsequently left the Christian Science Church and have lobbied against statutory religious exemptions to the child abuse and neglect laws.[3]

From the legal and medical perspective, the Christian Science community simply cannot be trusted by the dominant community to do what is best for their children without serious threats to the fundamental rights of these children. In the case of Robyn Twitchell, it seems clear to most physicians that respecting the beliefs and choices of Christian Scientists meant that Robyn's right to life and Robyn's right to minimally adequate health care were jeopardized. In a sense, respecting the wishes of these Christian Science parents meant that Robyn Twitchell was the subject of child neglect.[4] From the medical perspective, he may as well have been left alone by his parents to die, given what little his parents did to save his life. When the Twitchell case is used as a model, Christian Science seems to be the kind of community that cannot and should not be given equal respect with the other communities in our pluralistic society.

Consider another case of Christian Science refusal that is perhaps more representative of the clash between medical and Christian Science perspectives. In 1990, Colin Newmark's parents began to worry. The health of this three-year-old son of Christian Science parents had been deteriorating rapidly. The parents reluctantly took Colin to a hospital in Delaware near their home. The physicians could not immediately tell what was wrong with Colin and recommended extensive X rays and blood testing. The parents refused and took Colin home. Colin's condition continued to deteriorate and his parents returned to the hospital. X rays indicated that Colin suffered from an intestinal blockage. His parents agreed to surgery to remove the blockage, since they considered the procedure to be purely "mechanical."[5] "A pathological report on tissue taken from Colin's intestines during the surgery revealed that Colin was suffering from non-Hodgkins lymphoma. Five pathologists confirmed this diagnosis."[6]

The doctors in charge of Colin's case recommended chemotherapy and radiation that would give Colin a 40 percent chance of recovery. Without chemotherapy, the doctors argued that Colin would be dead in six to eight months. The form of chemotherapy proposed can result in kidney failure, hair loss, immunological and neurological problems, and, as a result of multiple blood transfusions, increased risk of infection. One of the doctors, Dr. Meek, "predicted that chemotherapy would bring Colin near death and that the radiation treatments required would presumably render him sterile."[7] The Newmarks rejected the chemotherapy and attempted to remove Colin from the hospital to be placed in the care of a Christian Science practitioner. The hospital sued to obtain custody of Colin in order to authorize the chemotherapy, and the hospital tried to have Colin placed into a foster home with caretakers who would cooperate with the medical treatment regimen. The Delaware Supreme Court sided with the Newmarks.

In many such cases it is not so clear that medical science can save the life of a child or that the side effects of saving the life are themselves not worse than the saving. We get a very different result if we use the model of Colin instead of that of Robyn in assessing the Christian Science refusal cases. The model of Colin is also consistent with the many children of Christian Scientists who seem to be quite healthy even though their parents don't accept medical authority. What is especially important about the case of Colin Newmark is that his parents did not blindly refuse to seek all forms of medical diagnosis and help. In the end they refused one form of proposed therapy, but such a refusal cannot seriously be said clearly to jeopardize Colin's fundamental rights. On the facts, it is not clear what would be best for Colin. Indeed, if this case had not concerned Christian Scientists, the medical profession would probably have been undivided in supporting, or at least not challenging, the parents' decision.

Christian Science

Since the Christian Science Church was founded over a century ago by Mary Baker Eddy, Christian Scientists have been locked in a struggle with the medical profession. In her major book, *Science and Health,* Eddy argues that "Mind," not matter, constitutes what is real. Each person should be able to be his or her "own physician, and Truth will be the universal panacea."[8] The power of prayer was thought to be an antidote to any ailment, since the ailments themselves were really mental in origin in the first place. In some cases, Eddy suggested that people may need help in bringing their minds into alignment with "Mind." Such help, in the form of reliance on certain others, was meant only to help the individual to help himself or herself.

Eddy formed a group of practitioners who were to aid individuals in finding mental or spiritual solutions to their problems. In the early years of the church, these practitioners were in direct competition with medical physicians. One recent writer on the history of these developments concludes as follows:

> Whereas osteopathy and chiropractic [the other dominant challengers to medical physicians at the turn of the century] followed the strategy of getting legislation passed that would govern their practices, Christian Science pursued the policy of obtaining amendments to the existing medical practice acts that specifically exempted its practitioners from their provisions. Thus, unlike the others who were regulated by the state, Christian Science was able to maintain complete administrative control over its practitioners.[9]

From the early years of the development of both the Christian Science and the medical communities, struggles between the two groups have been common.

According to Christian Science doctrine, children sometimes suffer material discomfort due to the mental beliefs of their parents. So the parents are sometimes in the best position to affect their children's health by bringing their own spiritual lives into order through prayer before the children's health will return.[10] Such a position does not seem to be at odds with seeking medical care for these children while the parents work on their spiritual well-being. But such is not the case, for Mary Baker Eddy comments that "hypocrisy is fatal to religion."[11] When Christian Scientists put their faith in spiritual healing, it is thought that it would be hypocritical also to put their faith in medicine. Some Christian Scientists fervently believe that the power of spiritual healing is greatly diminished if the faith of the person praying is so weak that medical help is sought at the same time that prayer is being made. Indeed, Eddy says that it "is a grave mistake to suppose . . . that Spirit and matter . . . can commune together."[12] And "if we trust matter, we distrust Spirit."[13]

Yet the Christian Science doctrine about the medical treatment of children is not as clear-cut as is sometimes supposed. There is no room in Christian Science for a blind faith in spiritual healing in all cases. "Nothing is more antagonistic to Christian Science than a blind belief without understanding," Eddy says.[14] And there is nothing in the doctrine to forbid anyone from seeking medical healing. Rather, there is a strong sense that someone who seeks medical healing has turned away from the power of spiritual healing. But even Eddy herself came, at the end of her life, to advocate seeking medical care during childbirth, and in *Science and Health* she allowed that surgery could be used to set broken bones.[15] Recently, the Christian Science board of directors issued a restatement of church policy. The statement said:

> Although it is entirely natural for students of Christian Science to rely on prayer, it is also important, when it comes to the care of children, that Scientists consider well their individual spiritual readiness, their own past experience and record, and the mental climate in which they live. . . . When circumstances result in a child's being brought under medical care, members of our Church would surely continue to cherish such a family and give them their full love and support during a challenging time. . . . To look upon another's progress with anything less than loving encouragement would not be Christian.[16]

Yet this restatement reaffirms that seeking medical care "clearly departs from the practice of Christian Science."[17]

These various nuances in the Christian Science doctrine, especially toward children, have resulted in a wide variety of Christian Science practices concerning sick children. The most interesting question from my perspective is why Christian Scientists have had such trouble seeing medical science as a diagnostic aid to their own attempts to remove disease through prayer. One reason for this may be that many Christian Scientists seem to take literally several passages in *Science and Health* (effectively the bible of Christian Science[18]) which say that little children should not be exposed to false belief and superstition, that is, to medical science. Using medical science as a diagnostic tool would be enough to give it credibility in the eyes of a child, which would diminish the authority of Christian Science and ultimately adversely affect the child, the family, and even the whole Christian Science community.

Yet, since even Mary Baker Eddy was willing to allow that Christian Science practices are not able to effectuate cures in all cases and that some "mechanical" forms of medical science should be relied on (i.e., as in the case of childbirth, broken limbs, and dentistry). Thus it seems odd indeed, even on the very principles of Christian Science and its emphasis on never accepting anything on blind faith, not to remain open to the possibility that more illnesses than those related to obstetrics, orthopedics, and oral surgery can be helped by medical diagnosis. At the very least, it would seem to make sense to know something about the physical condition of the body (even given that it is only effect and not cause of the illness) in order to be better able to direct one's spiritual resources.[19] The Christian Science response is to insist that medical diagnosis is potentially pernicious in two important ways. First, according to the metaphysical doctrine that undergirds Christian Science, illness is caused by such "mental," rather than physical, factors as how the person thinks about his or her bodily states. Since medical diagnosis is aimed at identifying what is wrong with the physical body, acceptance of such diagnoses could make it harder for the person to change his or her conception of the health of the body. Second, once a medical diagnosis has been rendered, it will be much harder for the Christian Scientist to retain control over the decisions concerning one's own health or the health of one's children. Past experience has shown, as in the case of Colin Newmark, that once physicians get a patient under their influence, they will try to force Christian Scientists to follow the medical regimen rather than the Christian Science one.[20] Medical diagnosis, so it is believed, can make things worse rather than better.

The official doctrine of the Christian Science Church opposes medical diagnosis,[21] but as I have been arguing, even Mary Baker Eddy found value in medical diagnosis in some cases. She distinguished between conditions that could be corrected by mechanical means and conditions (i.e., diseases) that could not. She remained opposed to diagnosis for disease, as has official Christian Science doctrine. It seems to me, though, that until diagnosis is performed, it isn't clear whether mechanical correction, something requiring medicine, or something even more invasive (such as surgery) is called for medically. If removing a bowel obstruction is mechanical, as some Christian Scientists seem to believe, then it would make sense to allow, even to encourage, diagnosis when symptoms of possible bowel obstruction manifest themselves, as well as in several other cases. But Christian Scientists have by and large remained committed to refusing any form of medical practice.

Medical Authority

Cases that involve the refusal of Christian Scientists to accept medical authority fall into two important groups: an adult who refuses treatment for himself or herself and a parent who refuses treatment for his or her child. In both cases, the medical establishment in the United States has opposed the refusal of medical care by Christian Scientists, and individual doctors have often responded with contempt and outrage to the public position of the Christian Science Church, namely, that the power of prayer is more effective than the power of surgery and medicine. It is clear that the medical establishment has not seen the refusal cases as simply a matter of conflicting beliefs but as a struggle for authority.

In the early part of the twentieth century, medical doctors consolidated their power and tried to enlist legal authorities in enforcing some of their decisions about what is best for patients, especially in life-threatening situations. Most adult Christian Scientists, especially in recent times, have managed to avoid what they perceive as the interventionistic strategies of medical doctors by simply staying clear of doctors and hospitals.

Many academics who work in medical ethics have recently broken ranks with their colleagues in medicine by arguing that adult Christian Scientists should be allowed to pursue matters of health on their own terms. Indeed, three well-known medical ethicists conclude a recent article on this subject with the following words: "The right of patients to forgo life-sustaining treatment has been well established in health law and medical ethics."[22] This change in consensus is due to the rejection of the doctrine of paternalism over the last twenty years.[23]

Many medical doctors strongly object to Christian Scientists who refuse treatment for themselves, but they save their strongest criticisms for Christian Scientists who refuse treatment for their children. Here the issue cannot easily be settled by reference to the doctrine of paternalism, for children cannot generally consent due to their lack of autonomy.[24] The general consensus among physicians is well stated by Norman Fost: "We're interested not just in the kids who die. What we're concerned about are the hundreds and hundreds more who suffer from inadequate medical treatment."[25] The medical community is nearly unanimous in condemning Christian Scientists who refuse treatment for their children.[26]

The American Academy of Pediatrics has recently been spearheading a movement to remove the religious exemption provisos to child neglect statutes throughout the United States.[27] This campaign is fueled by the belief that Christian Scientists and Jehovah's Witnesses should be forced to subject their children to the full range of curative powers at the disposal of modern medicine. The AAP's growing involvement in these legislative matters is fueled by the belief that child neglect and abuse are on the rise in the United States and need to be confronted.[28] The religious exemption is seen as a major impediment to the provision of the best of health care to all American children.[29]

Medicine in the United States is a profession in at least two senses of the term.[30] It embodies better than any other profession the idea of a group of people who all profess to be bound by a commitment to a particular ideal, roughly that which is found in the Hippocratic oath. And medicine is a profession in the sense that it is an organized institution that claims a considerable amount of authority for the judgments of its members. Over the last century, the medical profession in the United States has achieved the status of a virtual state-sanctioned monopoly. This means that the already enormous power and influence of medicine has been augmented by alliances with the legal profession.[31] This alliance is nowhere more apparent than in the Christian Science refusal cases. Nearly every medical or legal discussion of these cases has been critical of the Christian Science position.

The nearly unanimous voice of the medical profession in rejecting the Christian Science position stems from the common socialization of medical students in the United States. The Hippocratic oath and its "do no harm" dictum, as well as the general principle of beneficence, has been interpreted in such a way that medical students are trained to be quite aggressive in pursuing what they believe will be least harmful and most beneficial for their patients. Once a determination, or diagnosis, has been made, it is considered to be harmful for the patient not to acquiesce in the regimen prescribed to overcome the diagnosed illness or disease. A patient's refusal to follow the prescribed regimen is seen as a failure of the doctor, indeed a failure specifically in the sense that the aggressive pursuit of "do no harm" and patient benefit has not been fulfilled.

But there is another tradition in medicine that apparently has not been discussed as much in medical schools, at least until quite recently, as the dominant tradition I have just set out. This tradition can be traced back to Maimonides, who declared that "the physician should not treat the disease but the patient suffering from it."[32] This tradition has also found expression in the idea that physicians should treat their patients as persons.[33] At the moment I merely note the existence of this alternative approach, which, if made part of the common medical socialization, might produce a set of attitudes and practices that differ from the ones currently dominant in modern medicine.

Nonetheless, when patients challenge the authority of their physician this is perceived by the physician as an affront to his or her medical expertise and status as an authority. Because medicine has achieved a near monopoly over matters of health in the United States, the idea that there could be multiple authorities over matters of health is simply rejected out of hand. Medical science is conceived by physicians and lawyers alike to be the only legitimate way of promoting the health of the patient. Especially when the health of children is at stake, the medical and legal communities unite to preserve the authority of medicine in matters of health, even when the members of a religious minority challenge this authority.

Authority in a Pluralistic World

There has been a serious debate recently about the role of moral and political authority in a pluralistic world.[34] The term "authority" can be used in its "representation" sense as referring to someone who is given the ability to act or speak in behalf of another, or in its "expert" sense as referring to someone who is recognized simply to be more knowledgeable than most others in a certain domain of inquiry. One of the most important questions in the recent debate concerns whether these two senses should be merged so that those who have the most knowledge are, by that very fact, more legitimately able to act or speak on behalf of the rest of the population. In contemporary medicine, the physician's authority in terms of expertise is often transmuted into the physician's authority in terms of legitimacy to represent the community in determining how people should behave. One variation of this transmutation occurs when a medical doctor declares that he or she should have the right to decide what is in the best interest of a patient and to mandate that the patient follow the doctor's regimen toward securing that interest.

The exercise of authority by one person over another can restrict the freedom of the other. If the person over whom authority is exercised is a mature adult human being, then such exercise of authority may be illegitimate insofar as it restricts this person's autonomy.[35] The case of authority exercised over children does not normally raise the same problems, since children generally are not thought to have autonomy. Parents must be able to exercise some authority over their children in order to properly instruct and protect them. Until quite recently this parental authority was assumed to be nearly inviolable. This is a questionable assumption, since not all parents have the best interest of their children in mind, and some parents are quite mistaken about what is best for their children, or are even positively malicious, just as is true of certain members of nearly every group. Liberalism has traditionally placed very strong emphasis on individual rights to the exclusion of concern for the collective good of various groups. Various liberal theorists have talked of the rights of children, rights that are somewhat weaker than those of mature adults but are nonetheless strong enough to override the claims of various parents, families, or communities to act toward their children in ways that seem likely to lead to harm to these children.[36] Communitarians have been the most vociferous in arguing that traditional liberalism entrenches divisiveness and separateness, thereby making it difficult for groups, especially families, to achieve coherence and stability.

In pluralistic societies, there are multiple and overlapping social groups, indeed often so many groups with conflicting goals that it seems impossible to reconcile the claims of each. In such times it seems quite reasonable to focus on the individual rather than the group. But this is a mistake because often with the increase in isolation comes a loss of solidarity and an increase in rootlessness and alienation, especially among members of minority groups.[37] Ethnic, linguistic, and religious groups, when they exist as minority groups within a strongly dominant culture, need some protection from the larger community, which may engulf the minority culture at any time. Even in liberal societies minority rights have sometimes been trampled, especially the rights of religious minorities.

Charles Taylor has argued that there is a version of liberalism that would risk less harm to the collective goods and identity of minority groups. "A society with strong collective goals can be liberal, on this view, provided it is also capable of respecting diversity, especially when dealing with those who do not share its common goals; and provided that it can offer adequate safeguards for fundamental rights."[38] The Christian Science refusal cases offer a very good testing ground of Taylor's version of liberalism since, it is often claimed, the right of children to basic levels of health is precisely what is threatened by the collective goals of the Christian Science community. In addition, the Christian Science community's cohesiveness is thought to be threatened by the possibility that the medical community could force Christian Scientists to subject themselves to the power of the scalpel instead of the power of prayer.

The Christian Science refusal cases are better understood as a conflict between two communities (Christian Science and medical) than as a conflict between two individuals (Christian Science parent and medical physician). The seemingly irreconcilable nature of the positions in these cases is due to conflicting worldviews and conflicting conceptions of what counts as authoritative in matters of health; it is not merely a dispute about what should be done for a particular child. Physicians and Christian Scientists act as if much more is at stake than merely the health of a particular child. Indeed, Christian Scientists often talk as if the very future of their church hangs in the balance; and physicians often talk as if the very future of medical progress is at stake. This is why I think the issue is best addressed as a conflict of groups rather than as a conflict of individuals.[39]

The key question here is not only whether the physical health of a child is a fundamental right that should be given priority over such community goods as group cohesiveness but also whether the medical community should be given exclusive purview in determining what is best for securing that right. The difficulty is that the Christian Science and medical communities give very different, and seemingly incompatible, accounts of what is the best method to secure health. Is this sociopolitical clash of communities something that is subject to compromise, or must one community "win out," even in a pluralistic society? Taylor has claimed that "liberalism is not a possible meeting ground for all cultures, but is the political expression of one range of cultures, and quite incompatible with other ranges."[40]

Taylor is worried that even in a very diverse pluralistic society some groups may act in such a disruptive manner that they jeopardize the stability and coherence of the larger community. On this view, not all forms of authority can be challenged. Some limits must be placed, especially where the overall community's survival is at stake or where fundamental rights of individuals are threatened. His view is that only a certain range of cultural diversity can be sustained, and hence only certain minority cultures can be tolerated, in a particular political society. The range of toleration should be determined by whether any fundamental rights of individuals or groups are likely to be violated by a minority culture that is seeking full recognition and respect within the larger community.

I have argued in a similar vein that some sort of compromise between liberalism and communitarianism is needed.[41] I draw a distinction not only between fundamental and nonfundamental individual rights but also between systematic and occasional violation of these rights. Such a distinction is necessary, since there are many things that could jeopardize the fundamental rights of individuals that nevertheless do not constitute grounds for excluding the group that jeopardizes these rights. Consider, for example, the suspension of fundamental rights during a state of emergency. Arguably, the curtailment of a person's rights to free speech or press would normally be seen as a violation of fundamental individual rights. But this would not be sufficient to preclude this practice if the emergency were severe enough.

Most cultures risk the occasional violation of some fundamental rights. What normally cannot be tolerated is a minority culture that systematically jeopardizes a fundamental right of the members of the larger community. The Christian Science refusal cases do not show such systematic jeopardy of fundamental rights. In any event, the religious liberty of the members of these groups is of very high value, and in a pluralistic society it should be given strong weight. Of course, this is not to say, as some Christian Scientists have argued, that this issue can be decided simply on the grounds of religious freedom alone.

Seeking a Compromise

Today, the medical community and the Christian Science community continue to argue that all Christian Science refusal cases be treated alike. According to the American Academy of Pediatrics, neither Robyn Twitchell's nor Colin Newmark's parents should be allowed to refuse to accept medical authority. The position expressed by the AAP is hard to reconcile with the features of a pluralistic society. Although it is important to protect fundamental rights, Christian Science is not alone in occasionally jeopardizing the fundamental rights of individuals. But it is relatively alone in discouraging its members from seeking medical diagnoses. Such a stance may be a systematic risk to the fundamental rights of children. But it is not clear that Christian Scientists as a group should, on their own principles, discourage diagnosis. Indeed, the bylaws of the Christian Science Church state rather clearly that if "a member of this Church has a patient whom he does not heal, and whose case he cannot fully diagnose, he may consult with an M.D. on the anatomy involved."[42]

The compromise I propose involves two elements. Medical science should be more attuned to the whole person who is the patient, especially in non-life-threatening situations and hence to nonstandard approaches to health. Christian Science should be more open to the diagnostic services of medical science in order to ascertain what type of spiritual healing is needed so that informed decisions can be made about when to consider medical help, especially in life-threatening situations. For both of these elements to be achieved, the socialization practices of the medical and Christian Science communities must change so that their members do not see themselves as opposed to each other. Medical professionals should be more open to the possibility that there are at least some aspects of health that are not their sole purview. Christian Scientists should be more open to the possibility (seemingly admitted by Mary Baker Eddy) that there are aspects of health that are best dealt with by material (at least "mechanical") means.

This approach to resolving, at least temporarily, the stalemate between the Christian Science community and the medical community is more communitarian than liberal, since I remain committed to maintaining the coherence of these two communities.[43] The compromise that I propose is meant to be respectful to both of these communities. This is not to say that all of the members of the Christian Science and medical communities will find my approach acceptable. Indeed, I suspect that many members of these communities will reject it. But this just points out to what extent this is a compromise and not a consensus.

One standard way to think about the divide between liberalism and communitarianism is to think that liberals believe in compromise and communitarians believe in consensus. One of the paradigms of communitarianism is the Quaker meeting, and one of the paradigms of liberalism is deliberations in Congress. Yet, for consensus to be achieved in the Quaker meeting, many people will have to accept a compromise; and in Congress, the deliberative compromises often center on the common good. In light of these paradigms, I wish to propose that in pluralistic societies the move toward consensus sometimes denies or submerges differences among groups, and in this sense consensus runs contrary to communitarianism. Some compromises, on the other hand, really do leave group identities intact, since here both parties to a dispute temporarily must give a bit in order to achieve some higher social good.

The Christian Science refusal cases illustrate well the need to think in terms of compromise as well as consensus when conflicts arise among multiple authorities in a pluralistic society.[44] The rights of children, the authority of medicine, and the religious freedom of Christian Science must all be considered and balanced against each other. None of these factors should be considered overriding. Even a temporary solution to this problem will occur only when Christian Science and medical communities recognize that there are both Colin Newmarks, who may do better without medical intervention, as well as Robyn Twitchells, who may do better with that intervention.

My proposed compromise is likely to occur only when the medical community becomes willing to give Christian Scientists some room to consider the results of diagnostic testing without worrying that some doctor has already contacted a public prosecutor to force the Christian Scientists to accept proposed medical care. In addition, this change is only likely to occur when the Christian Science community stops discouraging its members from seeking medical diagnoses, and in life-threatening cases, seeking medical care. Just as the socialization practices of the medical community need to change so that its members are more open to the Christian Science community, so the socialization practices of the Christian Science community need to change so that its members are more open to the medical community. In the remainder of this essay I will consider three objections that could be raised against my view. In so doing, I will try to make more explicit the philosophical assumptions and reasonings that led me to propose the compromise.

Let us first consider the most serious problem with my proposed compromise. If there really is a metaphysical dispute separating medical and Christian Science communities, then neither side will be able to compromise without somehow giving in to the other side. If Christian Scientists really believe that, metaphysically, medicine cannot cure disease and that diagnosis somehow makes disease worse, then acknowledging that diagnosis is a good thing, or at least not something to be condemned, would cause Christian Scientists to give up on a major part of their worldview. And if medical scientists really believe that prayer can never cure, and that failure to diagnose and treat medically is tantamount to child neglect, then acknowledging that Christian Scientists should be allowed to pursue prayer rather than medical treatment would cause medical scientists to give up on a major part of their worldview.[45]

This first objection strikes at the very heart of my proposal, for it was my intent to show that neither party to this dispute would have to give up its worldview in reaching a compromise. I argued that Christian Scientists have, as far back as their founder Mary Baker Eddy, acknowledged the legitimacy of certain forms of medical treatment. And I argued that medical scientists have not been committed to pursuing physical health at the expense of the mental well-being of the patient. If I am right about this, then the worldviews, although conflicting on many points, are not completely at odds with each other. The key philosophical assumption that I make throughout the paper is that we should be respectful of the integrity of these communities. But being respectful does not mean allowing each community to set unreasonable demands on its members or on nonmembers. In deeply pluralistic settings, it is important not to let one community hold the members of another hostage over issues that are not of central concern.

This brings me to a second objection. It could be objected that Christian Scientists are not being reasonable about any of this, since they refuse to discuss the evidence upon which their claims for the power of prayer are based. Margaret Battin has argued at great length (in chap. 1) that Christian Scientists have tried to convince their members that the unexamined anecdotal evidence of cures based on prayer, rather than medicine, by church members is more important than the enormous amount of statistically significant data that modern medical science has amassed showing the curative power of medicine.[46] The fact that the Christian Science leadership has consistently refused to subject its claims about the power of prayer to critical scrutiny in anything like a double-blind test leads Battin to say that Christian Scientists are not deserving of respect for their views; rather, they are to be morally criticized for deluding their members.[47]

I have a lot of sympathy for some of what Battin says. It strikes me that the evidence cited by Christian Scientists is at best mushy. This is one reason for my urging them to at least consider medical diagnosis as a kind of second opinion about how to cure their children. The evidence supporting medicine's curative powers seems as overwhelming to me as it does to Battin. Yet it is also undeniable that in many cases medical science cannot identify the best strategy for curing a particular child. This is why cases such as the Newmark case should not be treated the same way as the Twitchell case. So, although I support the claim that Christian Scientists should be more open to testing the claims of efficacy of their curative methods, I do not think that their failure to do so means that they should be forced to accept medical authority in all cases. And I do not think that we should not respect this community even if it continues to resist critical scrutiny of its claims and methods of cure.

We now arrive at the third objection. It could be claimed that I have surreptitiously smuggled a major epistemological premise into my discussion. By construing the issue as one concerning conflicting perspectives or worldviews, each struggling for domination over the other, I have abandoned the possibility that there is a truth of the matter—some criterion by which we could independently assess these viewpoints and find them wanting. Calling the positions of Christian Science and medicine "perspectives" seems to suggest that each has equal standing and that to deny such equal standing is to fail to display equal respect for them. Conflicts between perspectives are seemingly claimed to be inevitable and irresolvable. Yet no argument is provided in favor of adopting this epistemological standpoint.[48]

It is true that I am at a loss in attempting to find an objective procedure for assessing the Christian Scientist's claims about the power of prayer. But I am not espousing a cultural perspectivalism. There are certain things that seem relatively uncontroversial, such as that it would have taken a very simple operation to remove the bowel obstruction from Robyn Twitchell and hence to save his life. But there are other things, such as that Robyn's life could also have been saved if people were to have prayed hard enough for him, that I would be hard pressed to deny even though I have a hard time believing it. I do not think that anyone really knows the truth about the power of prayer. If I am right, then it behooves us to adjust our laws so that we do not construct a presumption against those who rely on prayer rather than medicine. In a pluralistic democracy, especially where the truth of the matter is reasonably contested, laws should not be biased in favor of only one of two possible perspectives.[49]

Notes

1. My interest in this topic was fueled by many discussions with my fellow members of the St. Louis Children's Hospital Medical Ethics Subcommittee.

2. This is a paraphrase of an opinion voiced by the emergency room physician on call at the hospital to which Robyn was taken after death. Most of the details here are taken from Paula Monopoli, "Allocating the Costs of Parental Free Exercise: Striking a New Balance between Sincere Religious Belief and a Child's Right to Medical Treatment," *Pepperdine Law Review* 18 (1991): 323–324.

3. See Rita Swan, "Faith Healing, Christian Science and the Medical Care of Children," *New England Journal of Medicine* 309, no. 26 (1983).

4. The Twitchells' involuntary manslaughter conviction was overturned by the Supreme Judicial Court of the Commonwealth of Massachusetts in 1993, seven years after Robyn's death.

5. There is some dispute about this fact. The brief filed by Colin's parents when this case went to the Delaware Supreme Court asserts that the parents consented to this initial operation, at least in part, because of undue pressure from their doctor.

6. The facts of this case are taken from a case note on *Newmark v. Williams,* 588 A.2d 1108 (Del. 1991) written by Patrick Bouldin, which appeared in the *Journal of Family Law* 30 (1991–1992): 673–681, esp. 674. Colin Newmark is a pseudonym used by the Delaware courts to protect the privacy of the child and his parents.

7. Bouldin, *Journal of Family Law,* 675.

8. Mary Baker Eddy, *Science and Health with Key to the Scriptures* (1875; Boston: The First Church of Christ, Scientist, 1971), 144.

9. Norman Gevitz, "Christian Science Healing and the Health Care of Children," *Perspectives in Biology and Medicine* 34, no. 3 (Spring 1991): 425.

10. Eddy, *Science and Health*, 154.

11. Ibid., 7.

12. Ibid., 73.

13. Ibid., 234.

14. Ibid., 83.

15. See Norman Gevitz, "Christian Science Healing and the Health Care of Children," 427–428.

16. Christian Science Board of Directors, "Christian Scientists and the Practice of Spiritual Healing," *Christian Science Sentinel,* October 7, 1991, 25.

17. Ibid.

18. This is not to suggest that Christian Scientists do not also rely on the authority of the Old and New Testaments.

19. It should be noted that Mary Baker Eddy several times decries medical diagnosis for causing the very disease it seemingly diagnoses. See *Science and Health,* 161, 370.

20. I am grateful to Peggy DesAutels for helping me to see why some Christian Scientists have such a strong reaction against medical diagnosis.

21. I base this claim on various communications I have had with members of the central office of the Christian Science Church in Boston.

22. Stephen H. Miles, Peter A. Singer, and Mark Siegler, "Conflicts between Patients' Wishes to Forgo Treatment and the Policies of Health Care Facilities," *New England Journal of Medicine,* July 6, 1989, 48.

23. See Larry May, "Paternalism and Self-Interest," *Journal of Value Inquiry* 14, no. 4 (Fall/Winter 1980).

24. Of course, children vary greatly in maturity and in ability to understand complex issues, even children of roughly the same age. In any event, it is a mistake to lump all children together, treating the two-year-old in the same manner as the twelve-year-old.

25. Quoted in Ronald Munson's popular textbook, *Intervention and Reflection: Basic Issues in Medical Ethics,* 4th ed. (Belmont, Calif.: Wadsorth, 1992), 262.

26. In surveying recent work on this topic, I found only a couple of exceptions to this statement among the dozens of essays I read. The most notable exception was Norman Gevitz's article "Christian Science Healing and the Health Care of Children."

27. See Monopoli, "Allocating the Costs of Parental Free Exercise," 331.

28. See Norman Gevitz, "Christian Science Healing and the Health Care of Children," 429.

29. By the end of 1993, although three states—Hawaii, South Dakota, and Massachusetts—had changed their "state laws to remove language that allowed people to deny their children medical care for religious reasons . . . the majority of states [had] language that makes criminal prosecution difficult" (*New York Times,* December 19, 1993, 16).

30. For a fascinating discussion of this view, see the first chapter of Eliot Freid-

son's excellent study, *Profession of Medicine: A Study of the Sociology of Applied Knowledge* (New York: Dodd, Mead, 1970).

31. We should not ignore the other major alignment, namely, that between medical science and the enormous segment of the economy that is connected to medicine. Hospitals, drug companies, nursing homes, hospital suppliers, and so on constitute one of the largest sources of employment and economic activity in the United States.

32. As quoted in Emanuel Goldberger's book *How Physicians Think* (Springfield, Ill.: Charles C. Thomas, 1965), ix.

33. See Paul Ramsey's book *The Patient as Person* (New Haven: Yale University Press, 1970).

34. For a good general discussion of the various issues involved in this debate, see Richard De George's book *The Nature and Limits of Authority* (Lawrence: University of Kansas Press, 1985).

35. See Richard De George's helpful discussion of this issue in chapter 9 of his book *The Nature and Limits of Authority.*

36. For a good selection of positions on this issue, see William Aiken and Hugh LaFollette, *Whose Child? Children's Rights, Parental Authority, and State Power* (Totowa, N.J.: Littlefield, Adams, 1980).

37. See the discussion of this point in chapter 2, section 3, of Larry May, *The Socially Responsive Self* (Chicago: University of Chicago Press, 1996).

38. Charles Taylor et al., *Multiculturalism and the Politics of Recognition* (Princeton: Princeton University Press, 1992), 59.

39. Indeed, the rank-and-file individual members of these groups voice quite a bit of sympathy for the other. But in terms of the leadership of these groups—those who speak for the groups themselves—the situation looks hopeless.

40. Taylor, *Multiculturalism,* 62.

41. See the last chapter of *Sharing Responsibility,* by Larry May (Chicago: University of Chicago Press, 1992).

42. In *Church Manual of the First Church of Christ Scientist, in Boston, Mass.,* by Mary Baker Eddy (1895; Boston: The First Church of Christ Scientist, 1936), 47. Some Christian Scientists also cite *Science and Health,* 444, wherein Mary Baker Eddy says that one may temporarily take a medical approach to healing.

43. My use of the term "medical community" may be disputed. It is not completely clear that there is a coherent community here, especially in light of recent disputes between nurses and physicians about the future of health care. I am grateful to Bill McBride for pointing this out to me. I have in mind the community of physicians who have, as I have said, shown a surprising coherence on this issue.

44. See Martin Benjamin, *Splitting the Difference: Compromise and Integrity in Ethics and Politics* (Lawrence: University of Kansas Press, 1990).

45. I am grateful to Hamner Hill for forcefully articulating this objection in a commentary he presented on an earlier version of this chapter at the 1994 AMINTAPHIL meetings in Charleston.

46. See Battin's book *Ethics in the Sanctuary* (New Haven: Yale University Press, 1990). I am also grateful for the commentary that Battin provided on an earlier version of my paper at the 1994 AMINTAPHIL meetings in Charleston.

47. Kenneth Kipnis made a similar point in his commentary on an earlier ver-

sion of my paper presented at the 1994 AMINTAPHIL meetings in Charleston. Kipnis also raises serious questions about my construal of the legal issues, to which I will not respond here.

48. This objection was mounted by Kenneth Winston in private correspondence.

49. I am grateful to Peggy DesAutels for first stimulating my interest in this topic and patiently explaining some of the intricacies of the Christian Science position. She, of course, is not responsible for any misconstruals of the Christian Science position that remain.

6

Challenging Medical Metaphysics

Peggy DesAutels

In his discussion of Christian Science refusals of medical treatment, Larry May emphasizes the conflict between two groups—the medical establishment and Christian Scientists. He analyzes the legal and ethical issues arising from Christian Science refusal cases primarily from the perspective of a political philosopher. According to May, the issues at stake are embedded in the larger issue of how best to resolve the conflicts between groups over "moral and practical authority" within a pluralistic society. He proposes the following compromises between the two groups: (1) Members of the medical community should be socialized to be open to patients with alternative values and approaches to health, especially in non-life-threatening situations; (2) Christian Science parents should be socialized to take their children to medical doctors for medical diagnoses; and (3) when the children of Christian Science parents are diagnosed as having medically treatable life-threatening conditions, these children should be medically treated.

May is respectful of the Christian Science perspective, and his proposed compromise attempts in good faith to respond sensitively to a worldview very different from his own. I agree with May that the differences between the medical and Christian Science communities run deep. But unlike May, I think these differences and the practical conflicts that arise out of these differences are best analyzed first from a metaphysical perspective and *then* from an ethical perspective. Christian Scientists' values and behaviors stem directly from their beliefs about the nature of reality. Whether the two groups could or should compromise, and in what ways, can only be determined after one considers *equally* the belief systems of both Christian Scientists and the medical community. May's proposed compromise is biased in favor of the medical community because it is influenced by the secular materialist assumptions that he and the medical community share. I maintain that no compromise is needed. Rather, members of the two groups should respect each other's disparate world-views and health-related choices. In those rare situations in which a Christian Scientist consults with or obtains treatment from a medical professional, the medical professional should accommodate the Christian Scientist's wishes.

Like May, I serve as a medical ethicist on hospital ethics committees. But as a participant in these meetings, I have not experienced antagonism toward patients with unorthodox views. My experience is that many who serve on these committees have a genuine interest in understanding and accommodating divergent worldviews and value systems. This type of reaction is in line with the 1985 code for nurses provided by the American Nurses Association. It states that "individual value systems and life-styles should be considered in the planning of health care with and for each client."[1] Of course, this is easier said than done. I have also noticed that, in spite of good intentions, physicians and nurses are understandably limited in their ability to grasp and respond to views built on metaphysical assumptions that differ from their own. This is not surprising, given their choice of profession and the years of training involved in pursuing it.

Conflicts between Christian Scientists and medical professionals rest on significant disparities between religious idealist belief systems and secular materialist belief systems. Practical conflicts arise because medical professionals find it difficult (if not impossible) to respond appropriately to a worldview that challenges what they take for granted about "the way things are." The views held by Christian Scientists are (1) fundamentally different and (2) very much in the minority. As a result, they are neither understood nor taken seriously. Whenever a majority group oppresses a minority group, this oppression can take place without the dominant group's even realizing it. The minority group *must* understand, respond to, and defend itself against the "given" views and practices of the majority, but the dominant group can remain blithely unaware of and unresponsive to the views and practices of minority groups. This is especially true when minority views are religiously based, since it is assumed that matters of deep faith are not open to discussion. But in order for members of the medical community and the Christian Science community to have balanced and appropriate interactions with each other, the worldviews, value systems, and health-related practices of both groups must first be equally examined and understood.

A Conflict over Belief Systems

Medical science and the practices of medical professionals rest on secular materialist assumptions. Christian Science and the practices of Christian Scientists rest on religious idealist assumptions. Such opposing assumptions lead to and are embedded within incommensurable worldviews (see chap. 2). Larry May mentions that there are conflicting worldviews but stresses "conflicting conceptions of what counts as authoritative in matters of health" rather than conflicting metaphysical assumptions. Although the beliefs of most relevance to a Christian Scientist's health-related practices are those concerning the role of Mind (God) in healing, these beliefs are directly linked to other assumptions and commitments. As Martin Benjamin points out, the main elements of any worldview include deeply held commitments about the following:

1. God, that is, whether there is a God and, if so, what God is like;
2. the nature and purpose (if any) of the universe and human life;
3. the nature, justification, and extent of human knowledge and our capacity to acquire further knowledge; and
4. the basic nature of human beings (including, for example, their capacities for free will, goodness, compassion, selfishness, and, in certain worldviews, "sin" and "redemption").[2]

Obviously, a religious idealist's worldview is going to directly conflict with a secular materialist's worldview in relation to the commitments listed above. For secular materialists, there is no God. There is no ultimate purpose for life aside from one that humans create for themselves. Knowledge about reality is gained using the methods of science. Humans are bodies with brains. Minds are at best shimmering, illusory side effects of neuronal firings, for without brain-matter, there is no mind. When bodies die, both brains and minds die. A human life consists of whatever happens to a person in this world and ends when a person is no longer biologically alive.

For idealists, or more specifically, for Christian Scientists, God is infinite Mind. This "physical" world is merely a temporary illusion and matter is a shimmering side effect of mental forces and causes. Knowledge about reality is gained by such means as inspiration, spiritual insight, and living a life that harmonizes with God. What is real about human beings is eternal and spiritual. What is unreal about human beings is temporal and material.[3] God is viewed as infinite Mind, and all of God's creation is seen as expressing this Mind. Health, along with everything else, is conceived of in spiritual terms. Apparent physical conditions are healed by better understanding and demonstrating harmonious spiritual reality.[4] Such terms as "health," "disease," "healing," and even "diagnosis" refer ultimately to mental conditions and processes rather than bodily conditions and processes.

Christian Scientists value above all else a better understanding of God and God's ideas. This understanding is not just intellectual but is applied and demonstrated throughout a Christian Scientist's day-to-day experience. As the large number of published accounts of Christian Science healing shows, there is an apparent paradox at work here. Making spiritual well-being a first priority can result not only in improved emotional health but also in improved "physical" health.[5]

Many medical practitioners are themselves neither materialists nor idealists but are mind-body dualists who view themselves as consisting of both a material body and an immaterial soul. But this view contributes to the secular materialist perspective found within the medical community. Medical professionals train themselves and are considered to be the "experts" on issues relating to the health of the body; religious leaders (ministers, priests, rabbis) train themselves and are considered to be the "experts" on issues relating to the health of the soul. Because of this mind-body division of labor, the assumptions on which both medical science and the medical profession rest are secular materialist ones. A medical professional working within a materialist worldview will highly value keeping the body healthy (free of pain and functioning properly) in order to enable the patient to pursue happiness in *this* life. A patient living within a worldview containing religious idealist assumptions, however, will most value spiritual life—progressing in his or her understanding of spiritual reality. This spiritual progress is not necessarily tied to a healthy, pain-free body nor is it limited to life on earth.

The underlying conflict between medical professionals and Christian Scientists, then, is a metaphysical one that in turn leads to differing values, health-related concepts, and health-promoting practices. This is not to say that individual medical professionals who react negatively to Christian Scientists are reacting solely to a conflicting worldview. There could be a number of motivating factors involved. Certainly, May's point is well-taken that some physicians do not like to have their authority over health matters challenged. Others may be reacting simply to what they consider to be dangerous and neglectful health care practices. But they may react more strongly to this "neglect" by Christian Scientists than they would to more obvious neglect in low-income, undereducated families. There are relatively few Christian Scientists, but they are often well-educated, well-placed individuals who are indistinguishable by race and class from most medical professionals. As a result, Christian Scientists can be more threatening both because they "should know better" and because they have the intellectual and monetary means for convincing others to take their views and practices seriously.[6]

Christian Science and Children

Although metaphysical conflicts between the medical community and the Christian Science community run deep, both groups highly value the health of children. Both accept the norm that children be healthy, happy, and free from mental and physical suffering. The disagreement is over how this health is best conceived and achieved. In spite of May's attempt to take the beliefs and values of Christian Scientists into account, he steadfastly views the health of children and its best means of achievement from a medical perspective. He assumes that when push comes to shove (when a child has a life-threatening disease), medical diagnosis and medically proven treatments are best for a child.

As a starting point for his discussion and proposed compromise, May considers two "refusal cases" involving Christian Science parents. It is, of course, only from the medical perspective that a parent's choice *for* an alternative course of treatment is viewed as a "refusal." This is no small point. From the medical perspective, a "refusal of medical treatment" is viewed as a "refusal to do anything at all." I will return to a discussion of May's "refusal" cases. But in order to balance May's (and the medical community's) view, I provide what I term a "choosing Christian Science case."

Of course, no single case is capable of representing the wide range of situations and outcomes experienced by parents who choose to use a Christian Science approach to their children's health. Many Christian Science parents quickly and decisively address all conditions that arise, including those that appear life threatening, without ever needing to interact with the medical community. Only a very few parents, Christian Scientists included, face prolonged life-threatening conditions in their children. When children are seriously ill or injured, Christian Science and medically oriented parents alike must make difficult and soul-searching decisions that respond to the particulars of their situation. In the case described below, a mother is updated by medical professionals on her child's condition but relies exclusively on Christian Science to cure her child of a disease that is medically diagnosed as incurable.

Laurie Allard's parents were not Christian Scientists when she was born. Although she was taken to physicians many times during her childhood,

these physicians could neither diagnose nor treat Laurie's increasingly serious breathing difficulties. When Laurie was eleven years old, her mother,
Shirley Andrew Allard, was introduced to Christian Science. As she describes it, Shirley "readily embraced a mental change of base from the tran-
sient things of matter to the invariable, spiritual ideas of God." She spent
the next few years engaged in diligent prayer and study while homebound
with her daughter. Although Shirley gained a better understanding of
Christian Science during this time, Laurie became increasingly ill.

By the time Laurie was fourteen, a neighbor who was both a surgeon
and a friend expressed deep concern for Laurie's health. The Allards, in response to this concern, decided to again seek a medical diagnosis in order
to obtain, as Shirley puts it, "a deeper comprehension of the situation"
with which they were faced. This time Laurie was diagnosed as having
cystic fibrosis, and the Allards were told that Laurie's condition was both
incurable and terminal. The physicians on the case did not expect her to
live more than a month. Shirley Allard mentally countered both the diagnosis and prognosis with the spiritual view of reality that she now embraced
and continued treating Laurie using a Christian Science approach (without
medical treatment). Laurie's father, who supported the use of Christian
Science in this case but was not himself a Christian Scientist, did request
that Laurie continue with regular medical examinations. These periodic
examinations were continued.

Shirley Allard dedicated herself even more completely to a course of prayer
and study. She describes one of the changes in her approach: "From then on,
every time her [Laurie's] condition was 'updated' on visits to the medical
specialist, I worked specifically to reverse, through prayerful treatment, whatever was predicted or diagnosed." She goes on to describe the turning point
that took place one evening in her own thought and in her daughter's health
when she "knew with all of [her] heart that God did not see [her] daughter
as a little bag of bones—disabled and frail—lying in a bed, but as His very
daughter, His perfect likeness." She went to bed "knowing that the facts
were as He saw them and that He forever sees what He has made."[7] For the
first time in many years, both she and Laurie slept through the night. It was
after this deeply experienced insight about God's and Laurie's real nature
that Laurie began to improve and then to thrive. She soon was entirely cured
of cystic fibrosis, using only a Christian Science approach. The published account concludes with brief verifying comments from Laurie herself, Laurie's
father, and a physician who asked that his name be "withheld."[8]

My point in retelling this case is to show that it cannot be assumed by
May or anyone else that a Christian Science approach will be ineffective in

the treatment of life-threatening diseases in children. This is just one published account among thousands of very serious conditions being completely healed using Christian Science. At the very least, medical professionals should acknowledge how little they understand about the relation of mind to body and should not assume that a spiritual approach to the healing of life-threatening illnesses is equivalent to "doing nothing." At best, they should respect and support those parents who are deeply committed to a spiritual approach to healing. Just as in the Allard case described above, when medical professionals and Christian Scientists do interact, they can do so cooperatively and without conflict.

Christian Science and Compromise

Although Christian Scientists may choose to seek medical information (as in Laurie Allard's case), in most health-related situations, they do not. May proposes that the Christian Science community compromise with the medical community by making medical diagnoses the rule rather than the exception, and he offers several reasons why more diagnoses would benefit Christian Scientists. At one point, he argues that even when Christian Scientists use their own approach, they would only benefit from knowing more about the physical condition of the body. At another point, May reasons that Christian Scientists would benefit from being informed of what procedures are called for medically, presumably including the "certain" dire consequences of refusing to submit to these procedures, in order to avoid "blindly" using Christian Science. Finally, May reasons that Christian Scientists should obtain more medical diagnoses so they can avoid death by switching to a medical approach when diagnosed with medically treatable life-threatening conditions.

Let us first examine May's suggestion that a Christian Science approach can (and therefore should) incorporate obtaining a medical diagnosis. Although May briefly mentions a few of the reasons why Christian Scientists avoid obtaining medical diagnoses, he does not view them as good reasons. For example, May does note that one reason Christian Scientists avoid obtaining medical diagnoses is due to their belief that disease is caused by mental rather than physical factors. Nonetheless, he asserts that even from the Christian Science perspective "it would seem to make sense to know something about the physical condition of the body (even given that it is only effect and not cause of the illness) in order to be better able to direct one's spiritual resources." But Christian Scientists would actually compromise their worldview by focusing on the physical condition of the body. When ill, they attempt to turn their attention away from the physical evidence in order better to focus on the harmonious spiritual nature of the situation. Christian Scientists view disease as ultimately an error in thought correctable only by an increased understanding of spiritual reality. May, on the other hand, thinks that this view needs to be supplemented by the "real" view of disease as material and treatable only by material means—that Christian Scientists are blind to the *actual* nature of a situation until they are given the medical perspective.[9] The bias here is clear. May does not suggest that the medical community would and should be benefited from learning more about how Christian Scientists view disease and its treatment.

May also fails to acknowledge some of the more important harms that can come from seeking medical diagnoses. Regardless of whether or not a patient is a Christian Scientist, the process of obtaining a medical diagnosis is certainly not the neutral, let alone always beneficial, process that May appears to think that it is. Steps and missteps involved in determining the name of a disease can include numerous visits to various physicians and specialists; invasive and painful tests and procedures; and "best guesses" that can turn out to be misdiagnoses. A significant number of internal conditions are medically diagnosable only by exploratory surgery. The invasive, painful, and potentially harmful procedures involved in obtaining diagnoses are enough for many non-Christian Scientists to avoid obtaining them whenever possible.

Of special significance to Christian Scientists, however, is the fact that much more happens in a physician's office than ordering diagnostic procedures. Because physicians firmly believe that certain conditions are *medical* conditions that are only treatable medically, they will push the patient to accept the reality of a medical condition, will describe the dire consequences of refusing their prescribed regimens, and will usually either subtly or overtly try to coerce the patient into undergoing medical treatment. In such situations, whereas the doctor "agrees" with the disease and its predicted course, the Christian Scientist "disagrees" with the disease and mentally argues against its legitimacy in her experience as part of her prayerful response. Whereas the doctor looks for and describes a material cause of the disease, the Christian Scientist looks for the cause in thought and seeks to address it through a better understanding of her Godlike, spiritual nature. The doctor believes that only medical interventions can cure certain diseases; the Christian Scientist believes that only an improved understanding of spiritual reality can address the underlying causes of disease. Why would a Christian Scientist choose to initiate a direct conflict with a physician over beliefs about the nature of disease, its causes and cures?

Even many non-Christian Scientists have become concerned over recent pressures from the medical community to "medicalize" many emotional patterns, addictive behaviors, and what are quite arguably normal variations in bodily states. Patients are encouraged to view themselves as diseased, surrender responsibility for their conditions, and submit to medical "treatments." May does not acknowledge the need for some patients to resist this pressure and to view themselves as healthy when physicians view them as sick. His stance leaves room for physicians to deem incompetent those Christian Science patients who "do not understand" medical diagnoses and prognoses. May does acknowledge that Christian Science patients are at risk of being coerced by physicians into following medical regimens, and he ostensibly encourages physicians to remain open to their patients' use of alternative approaches. Nevertheless, May recommends that Christian Science patients submit to medical authority concerning both the nature of their physical conditions and the prognoses for their conditions when left medically untreated. Some of the most obvious reasons for Christian Scientists to avoid obtaining medical diagnoses, then, are to avoid the need to resist much that physicians describe and prescribe and to avoid being deemed incompetent when they do resist.

May correctly notes that the doctrine of Christian Science contains no hard-and-fast behavioral rules about seeking medical diagnoses. The Christian Science Church is not authoritarian about the behavior of its members, nor does it threaten excommunication or damnation if a Christian Scientist chooses to seek a medical approach. Christian Scientists are given guidance on how to approach health-related matters but are expected to make autonomous choices. Just because the church "allows" diagnoses does not mean that there are no good reasons for Christian Scientists to avoid obtaining them. Nor does it mean that there is justification for coercing or even "socializing" Christian Scientists into obtaining them.[10]

Every once in a great while Christian Scientists or Christian Science practitioners may decide that knowing the name of a particular condition would aid their healing efforts.[11] They may even decide, in such cases, that the potential benefits of consulting a physician for a diagnosis outweigh the potential harms. But this is rare. In most cases, the name of the condition is already suspected if not known, and in those cases where it is not, the patient at least knows what condition is most *feared*. Christian Scientists find that prayer devoted to addressing and allaying this fear usually results in the symptoms disappearing without ever needing to consult a physician about the name of a condition. Seldom would a Christian Scientist who is using

a Christian Science approach to healing view the potential benefits of obtaining a medical diagnosis to be greater than the potential harms.

May stresses what he considers to be the benefits of medical *diagnoses*
for Christian Scientists because he is aware that a Christian Scientist who
has chosen a Christian Science approach to treating an illness would not
(with very few exceptions) consider medical *treatment* to be compatible
with that approach. But a large part of why May advocates socializing
Christian Scientists to seek more medical diagnoses is so that they can opt
for medical treatment when they are diagnosed with life-threatening conditions. May thus recommends not only that Christian Scientists encourage each other to switch to an approach that conflicts with their own but
also that they switch to this approach whenever the *medical community*
deems a condition to be life threatening. May appears to make the following assumptions: (1) Conditions diagnosed by a physician as life threatening cannot be treated successfully using a Christian Science approach, (2)
some types of life-threatening conditions are *easily* treated using a medical
approach, and (3) when a life-threatening condition is "easily" treated
medically, then a patient *should* choose that treatment.

There are obvious problems with all three of these assumptions. First,
the large body of published accounts of Christian Science healing includes
many cases that were medically diagnosed as life threatening or terminal.
So at least some Christian Scientists have fully recovered from some "life-
threatening" diseases without the use of medical means. Second, few medical treatments of life-threatening conditions are without risk and/or
serious side effects. Much as medical professionals downplay them, there
are always risks: adverse reactions to medications, infections from surgery,
contracting diseases to which a patient is exposed during a hospital stay,
professional ineptness, and so on. It is significant, also, that usually the risks
of harm from treatment are proportionate to both the seriousness of the
condition and the invasiveness of the treatment. Third, no patient—
Christian Scientist or anyone else—is morally obligated to choose to have
medical treatment regardless of how "simple" the medical community considers the treatment to be.[12] Whether to treat a condition and with what
approach should be a matter of individual conscience.

Christian Scientists and Accommodation

Up to this point, I have stressed the reasons Christian Scientists have for
avoiding both medical diagnoses and medical treatments. But there are
times when Christian Scientists are willing to accommodate the needs and

worries of others within their larger community. The most obvious is when Christian Scientists exhibit symptoms of an infectious disease. If a particular disease is of concern to their community, Christian Scientists willingly report their symptoms to the appropriate health officials. They also quarantine themselves when it is requested and obtain vaccinations when it is required.

In general, Christian Scientists do care about and are responsive to the concerns and fears of those with whom they interact. They recognize that some medically oriented members of society can be quite alarmed when their Christian Science colleagues, neighbors, or loved ones choose a non-medical approach to "medical" conditions. Because society is especially focused of late on the well-being of children, most Christian Science parents are particularly aware of the need to proceed thoughtfully and carefully when making health-related choices for their children. As May points out, Christian Scientists have received a communication from the Christian Science board of directors recommending that "when it comes to the care of children, . . . [Christian] Scientists [should] consider well their individual spiritual readiness, their own past experience and record, and the mental climate in which they live."

Perhaps the most instructive types of accommodations are those that take place when one parent is a Christian Scientist and the other is not. Such "dual-approach" parents vary widely in how they reach health care decisions for their children, but normally each parent has at least an equal respect for and a minimal understanding of the worldview of the other. Under such conditions, often the non-Christian Science parent gives the Christian Science parent the first opportunity to address a child's health problem. If the child does not improve within an agreed-upon time frame, the child is then taken to see a physician. Only when the condition is not addressed adequately using Christian Science is a medical approach used. Notice that in this kind of give-and-take, the parents do not attempt to compromise by using both a Christian Science approach and a medical approach *at the same time*. If this kind of accommodation is to be called a "compromise," the compromise is diachronic rather than synchronic.

Even when both parents are Christian Scientists, it is in accordance with Christian Science teachings and an expectation within the Christian Science community that a child be healed and not be allowed to suffer. What is at issue, however, are the conditions under which Christian Science parents make the determination that their preferred approach of Christian Science treatment is not working. Even for those parents who are not Christian Scientists, society has no clear norms on when a child should be taken to a physician. Some parents take a child in for the slightest scrape or sniffle. Others recognize that most childhood illnesses are self-limiting and that there is usually little that a physician can do. Christian Science parents, along with many non-Christian Science parents, recognize that visits to physicians are seldom necessary for the day-to-day health of their children. And because Christian Science parents do not view themselves as "doing nothing," they will often choose to continue using a spiritual approach for a child even when many medically oriented parents would take a child in. As long as a child is not suffering unduly and appears to be responding positively to prayer, a Christian Scientist considers the potential benefits of sticking with a Christian Science approach to outweigh the potential harms of a medical approach. These benefits include healing without side effects and the gaining of highly valued spiritual insight that comes from meeting a challenge through prayer.

Just as non-Christian Science parents (and even physicians) can make mistakes in judgment over the severity of a child's condition, so too can some Christian Science parents. But only hindsight is twenty-twenty, and it is not fair that the reasonable mistakes in judgment made by Christian Science parents are prosecuted in courts and remarkably similar mistakes made by more medically oriented parents or by family physicians are not.

Let us reexamine one of the "refusal" cases discussed by May. Although David and Ginger Twitchell's conviction of involuntary manslaughter was overturned on appeal, May describes this case as one that "most doctors and lawyers take to be a good illustration of why we should not recognize the authority of Christian Science parents or give equal respect and treatment to the Christian Science community."

In his brief summary of the events leading up to the death of two-year-old Robyn Twitchell, May describes Robyn as experiencing five days of "intense pain and vomiting" prior to dying of what was later determined to be a bowel obstruction. May asserts, "What makes the case of Robyn Twitchell so tragic is that a relatively simple operation could have saved his life. The fact that his parents refused even to secure a medical diagnosis meant that they were completely unaware of how seriously ill their son was." Certainly Robyn's death—a death unintended and unexpected by his parents—was tragic. But I maintain that the choices made by Christian Scientists are often caricatured by those holding to a conflicting perspective. When the specifics of this case and others like it are examined, the parents are not so obviously culpable as May and the medical community make them out to be.

According to the brief of appellants David and Ginger Twitchell (*Commonwealth of Massachusetts v. David R. Twitchell and Ginger Twitchell*), the events leading up to Robyn's death were as follows:

In April 1986, after a five-day intestinal illness, two-and-a-half-year-old Robyn Twitchell suddenly died. The first sign of his illness appeared in the middle of the night when he awakened crying and in apparent pain. His parents, defendants David and Ginger Twitchell, asked "if it hurt" and Robyn pointed to his tummy. Sometime thereafter he vomited.

From that episode in the small hours of a Friday morning through the following Tuesday evening, Robyn's condition fluctuated. He showed symptoms of illness alternating with signs of apparent recovery. During some periods, Robyn showed such symptoms as pain, vomiting, loss of appetite, drowsiness, or lethargy. At other times, eyewitnesses found him playful, alert to his environment, interested in food, and while not "feeling 100%," not "seriously ill." On Tuesday, he seemed remarkably better during the day. But in the evening, he took a final turn for the worse and, to the astonishment and lasting grief of his parents, suddenly passed away in his father's arms.

An autopsy found that Robyn died of an obstructed bowel that had twisted and untwisted around a fibrous band associated with a rare congenital anomaly known as Meckel's diverticulum. Such twisting and untwisting can produce corresponding signs of illness and recovery until the twist becomes fixed. On Tuesday, Robyn's bowel perforated, releasing intestinal pressure and producing a false sense of recovery—while quickly bringing on fatal peritonitis.

During those five days, Robyn's parents, defendants David and Ginger Twitchell, tended to him faithfully. They held him, comforted him, slept beside him. And as devout Christian Scientists, they sought healing for their son through the spiritual treatment that is the distinguishing feature of that faith. They availed themselves of help from every kind of support person in the Church service system. They retained a Christian Science Practitioner, Nancy Calkins, who a week earlier had successfully healed what appeared to be a similar intestinal illness in Robyn's older brother, Jeremy. They also employed a Christian Science nurse, and consulted a person associated with the Mother Church. When Robyn experienced significant periods of relief, the Twitchells felt confident that he was improving under spiritual care. As his symptoms recurred, however, they knew that healing remained incomplete.[13]

I submit that the parents in this case are no more morally culpable than any other parents or physicians who, unaware of the severity of the situation, continue in good faith with a healing approach that has worked for them in the past and appears to be working for them now.

One can easily imagine Robyn's case turning out similarly with parents who are not Christian Scientists. A child was vomiting one week after an older child had intestinal flu. The symptoms were a little different, but many parents recognize that children can experience illnesses differently. If a physician had been called early on, a variation of intestinal flu may well have been diagnosed. When the child failed to improve after a few days, if the child had then undergone more diagnostic procedures, the child *may or may not* have been correctly diagnosed as having Meckel's diverticulum. Several diseases mimic this condition, including such self-limiting diseases as gastroenteritis.[14] Finally, if Meckel's diverticulum had been correctly diagnosed and corrective surgery performed, the child *may or may not* have survived the surgery let alone thrived. Although May trusts a physician who claims that Robyn's condition "could have been readily corrected by surgery with an almost one hundred percent chance of success," researchers who studied over two hundred cases of Meckel's diverticulum estimate morbidity from corrective surgery to be as high as 12 percent.[15]

It *is* tragic when children die because of mistakes in judgment or treatments that fail. But honest mistakes made by the Twitchells while using an approach that previously worked for them (and for thousands of others like them) are no more immoral than the mistakes and failings made by those using a dominant but nonetheless fallible medical approach. It is worth noting here that the child who starred in the movie *Poltergeist* died from the same condition after being misdiagnosed by her physician as having the flu.

An Alternative "Compromise"

The medical community and the Christian Science community can interact with each other in mutually beneficial ways. But I see no reason to compel the Christian Science community to compromise with the medical community in ways that Christian Scientists deem harmful to their well-being. Just as I do not insist that the medical community be compelled to incorporate the worldview and practices of Christian Scientists, I deny that Christian Scientists should be compelled to incorporate the worldviews and practices of the medical community. I do suggest that Christian Scientists take special care to notice when and if a Christian Science approach is not working in the case of children. Because members of the medical community are understandably biased by their own worldview, the final determination of when Christian Science parents should switch to a medical approach should *not* be left to members of the medical community. And in those rare cases in which Christian Science parents do make tragic mistakes in judgment, they should not be held more morally and legally responsible than any other parents or physicians who make similar tragic mistakes.

The worldview of medical professionals is the dominant one in our society. Members of the medical community need to understand that some alternative approaches to health are derived from worldviews that challenge and conflict with their own. Ideally, medical training would include a healthy dose of philosophy of medical science. As part of this dosage, medical students could and should be exposed to the assumptions embedded in the worldview of their profession and to possible alternatives to these assumptions. There is little that medical professionals can claim as "proven fact" regarding the causes of a particular patient's mental and physical symptoms. Alternative worldviews and their accompanying approaches to treating illness can and do work for those people who hold to and live within these worldviews.

I propose that when, for whatever reasons, a Christian Scientist seeks medical diagnosis or treatment, interactions between the Christian Scientist and the medical professional start from a basis of mutual respect. If a Christian Science parent brings a child to a doctor for medical diagnosis but wishes to continue to use a Christian Science approach, the medical professional should respect that parent's wishes. The medical professional should give the Christian Scientist room to use a Christian Science approach without interference even when the medical professional is "sure" (from a medical perspective) that the approach will not work. If a Christian Scientist decides to switch to a medical approach, medical professionals should continue to confer with the Christian Scientist over how much treatment to administer and for how long.

Because the worldview of Christian Scientists is a minority one, members of the Christian Science community do not need to be further educated on the dominant secular materialist worldview of medical science. They are culturally immersed in it. Nonetheless, there are some ways that Christian Scientists can and should facilitate appropriate interactions with medical professionals. Certainly, a Christian Scientist's health care decisions should not arise from undue fear of medical professionals and settings. Nor should they arise from an unbending rigidity that fails to take into account the progress (or lack thereof) of Christian Science treatment, the surrounding community's concerns, and so on. Christian Science is not a fundamentalist religion, and Christian Scientists should be alert to avoiding any fundamentalism in the Christian Science culture.

Notes

1. *Code for Nurses with Interpretative Statements* (Washington, D.C.: American Nurses Association, 1985).

2. Martin Benjamin, *Splitting the Difference: Compromise and Integrity in Ethics and Politics* (Lawrence: University of Kansas Press, 1990), 88.

3. Mary Baker Eddy, the founder of Christian Science, summarizes this view in "The Scientific Statement of Being" on page 468 of *Science and Health with Key*

to the Scriptures: "There is no life, truth, intelligence, or substance in matter. All is infinite Mind and its infinite manifestation, for God is All-in-All. Spirit is immortal Truth. Matter is mortal error. Spirit is the real and eternal. Matter is the unreal and temporal. Spirit is God, and man is His image and likeness. Therefore, man is not material. He is spiritual."

4. As Mary Baker Eddy puts it, "When the illusion of sickness or sin tempts you, cling steadfastly to God and His idea. Allow nothing but His likeness to abide in your thought. Let neither fear nor doubt overshadow your clear sense and calm trust, that the recognition of life harmonious—as Life eternally is—can destroy any painful sense of, or belief in, that which Life is not" (*Science and Health,* 495).

5. From 1969 to 1988, the *Christian Science Journal* and the *Christian Science Sentinel* published over 7,000 accounts of healing. Of these, 2,337 were healings of medically diagnosed conditions. Diagnosed conditions healed using a Christian Science approach include malignancy or cancer (including bone cancer, lymph cancer, skin cancer, cancer of the liver, breast, intestine, and uterus), tumor, polio, tuberculosis, pneumonia (including double pneumonia), heart disorders, kidney disorders, broken bones, childbirth complications, meningitis, appendicitis (some acute), scarlet fever, rheumatic fever, cataract, diabetes (including a juvenile case), pernicious anemia, rheumatoid or degenerative arthritis, gangrene, glaucoma, hepatitis, leukemia, multiple sclerosis, blindness, goiter, curvature of the spine, epilepsy, crossed eyes, and cleft palate. See *An Empirical Analysis of Medical Evidence in Christian Science Testimonies of Healing, 1969–1988* (Boston: Committee on Publication, The First Church of Christ, Scientist, 1989).

6. Christian Scientists have been quite effective, for example, at making their case to state legislatures, appealing to insurance companies to cover the costs of Christian Science treatment, and even at producing a well-respected newspaper.

7. Shirley Allard, "Report of Healing," *The Christian Science Journal,* June 1992.

8. It is worth noting that a physician can feel at risk verifying a nonmedical cure even when an effective medical treatment is unavailable.

9. May actually uses the term "blindly" when he refers to Christian Scientists who "blindly refuse to seek all forms of medical diagnosis and help."

10. Because Christian Science is neither fundamentalist nor authoritarian in nature and because there are no "punishments" for Christian Scientists who use medical treatment, it has been difficult to convince the courts of the burdens of medical treatment on the free exercise of religion for Christian Scientists. In *Walker v. Superior Court,* the court justified state regulation of Christian Science parents because it did not consider the burden of medical treatment on Christian Science religious practice to be that great. The court reasoned that "resort to medicine does not constitute 'sin' for a Christian Scientist, does not subject a church member to stigmatization, does not result in divine retribution, and, according to the Church's amicus curiae brief, is not a matter of church compulsion." See Deborah Sussman Steckler, "A Trend toward Declining Rigor in Applying Free Exercise Principles: The Example of State Courts' Consideration of Christian Science Treatment for Children," *New York Law School Law Review* 36 (1991): 499.

11. One aspect of prayer in Christian Science is to mentally "argue" against the

claim(s) of a particular disease. Mary Baker Eddy includes the following statement in *Science and Health:* "To heal by argument, find the type of the ailment, get its name, and array your mental plea against the physical" (p. 412).

12. As Richard DeGeorge notes in his own comments on an earlier version of May's essay, "Despite what anyone may think of the wisdom of their views, I have seen no argument to the effect that Christian Scientists (or anyone else) can be forced to visit a doctor when they have physical problems, that they must listen to doctors, follow their prescriptions, take the medicine they prescribe or allow them to operate. Any person may refuse, and the Christian Scientist is in no special position in this regard." (*Hastings Center Report,* May–June 1995, G1.)

13. *Commonwealth of Massachusetts v. David R. Twitchell and Ginger Twitchell,* no. SJC-06115, Brief of Appellants David and Ginger Twitchell.

14. The most common symptom of Meckel's diverticulum in childhood is bleeding. See Courtney M. Townsend Jr. and James C. Thompson, "Small Intestine," in *Principles of Surgery,* ed. Seymour I. Schwartz, M.D., G. Tom Shires, M.D., and Frank C. Spencer, M.D., 5th ed. (New York: McGraw-Hill), 1212. In comments on Meckel's' diverticulum on the Internet, one patient mentioned suffering intermittent abdominal pain for over nine months before physicians correctly diagnosed the condition.

15. See M. J. Soltero and A. H. Bill, "The Natural History of Meckel's Diverticulum and Its Relation to Incidental Removal: A Study of 202 Cases of Diseased Meckel's Diverticulum Found in King County, Washington, over a Fifteen-Year Period," *American Journal of Surgery* 132 (1976): 168. Comments on the Internet from people who have had corrective surgery for Meckel's diverticulum include patients who continue to have significant health problems following surgery, including chronic abdominal pain and diarrhea.

7

Respecting Medical Science and Christian Science

Larry May

Peggy DesAutels raises a number of interesting points in her response to my chapter on the Christian Science refusal cases. She rightly begins by noting that various codes of ethics for health care professionals call for sensitivity to minority members who may have beliefs and values that are quite different from those of the health care professional. As DesAutels reminds us, the 1985 code for nurses of the American Nursing Association says that "individual value systems and life-styles should be considered in the planning of health care with and for each client." My dispute with DesAutels turns on what it means for a health care professional to give serious consideration to the value systems of minority members who are their patients.

DesAutels endorses the view that the minority religious value systems should be given overriding weight over any decisions by health care professionals. Specifically, she says, "Where a Christian Scientist consults with or obtains treatment from a medical professional, the medical professional should accommodate the Christian Scientist's wishes." My position is that sensitive health care professionals need to give the beliefs and values of minority religious patients a lot of consideration in their deliberations, but such consideration falls short of having overriding weight in these deliberations. I feel the same way about the medical scientists; their views should not be given overriding weight either. My compromise solution tried to counter the overriding weight view, whether it comes from Christian Scientists or medical scientists.

In this brief response I defend the compromise I outlined in chapter 5 by showing that it does demonstrate respect for the values of patients. First,

I explain why the strong "overriding weight" view is implausible by considering a case of a religion that includes a ritual of human sacrifice. Second, I argue that DesAutels mischaracterizes what is at stake between medical science and Christian Science, specifically, she overestimates the importance of metaphysics. Third, I dispute DesAutels's claim that urging Christian Scientists and medical personnel to change the way their members are socialized amounts to coercion. Fourth and finally, I argue that it would be a mistake to give either the parents of Christian Science children or medical personnel overriding weight in regard to decisions made on behalf of sick children who cannot yet express their own views about either religion or medicine.

The Overriding Weight View

Let us begin by considering a religion with views that are much more unorthodox than those of Christian Science: Every year one prepubescent member of the religious community is sacrificed to the gods of this religion by being set ablaze upon the altar of their main church at midnight on their holiest of days, October 31.[1] Using DesAutels's criteria, we should give overriding weight to these people because they hold views that differ fundamentally from the majority view of members in their society, and as a result they are not understood or taken seriously by the majority. The question for us to consider is whether the sincerity of these beliefs and the fact that they are minority beliefs should grant them a status so high that they could justifiably override attempts by the majority community to protect the children of this religion from being killed.

It seems obvious to me that we should answer this question in the negative. Even in pluralistic societies, not all views can be tolerated. If we are to be persuaded by DesAutels, we will need additional arguments from her than the simple intuitive insight that minority religious members need to be protected from the tyranny of the majority. She sometimes says that the members of the majority need to give equal concern and respect to minority religious views. But what precisely does this amount to? In the case of the religion with the ritual of child sacrifice, would it be disrespectful of their religion to try to convince these people to stop this practice? DesAutels indicates that Christian Scientists should not be coerced to accept lifesaving medical care for their dying children. How would she distinguish the Christian Science case from the child sacrifice case? She either needs to explain much more about the meaning of respect, so that she can show that it would be respectful to intervene in the one but not the other case, or she needs to bite the bullet and extend her argument to countenance religiously motivated child sacrifice.

It is not intuitively obvious to me that respect or consideration for the beliefs and values of a religious minority means giving overriding weight to those beliefs and values, which is not to say that Christian Scientists can justifiably be coerced into accepting what the majority thinks is the right thing to do with their sick children. But it does mean that DesAutels has a harder job than she seems to realize in establishing the truth of the overriding weight view in respect to the health needs of sick Christian Science children. I will return to this point in the final section of this chapter. I now turn to one of DesAutels's most intriguing arguments for thinking that the general dispute between Christian Scientists and medical scientists is intractable and beyond the possibility of compromise.

The Relevance of Metaphysics

DesAutels claims that modern medicine rests on a view she calls "secular humanism," which has as one of its beliefs that "there is no God." As a result she then claims that the dispute between Christian Scientists and medical scientists is primarily a metaphysical dispute and for that reason a dispute that it will be nearly impossible to adjudicate. It is an inference of this view that we need to be deeply respectful of each of these views; their metaphysical assumptions are so different that their adherents simply cannot understand each other. I am sympathetic to some of what she says here, but I think she misstates the basis of medical science and hence makes the dispute seem more intractable than it is.

It is certainly true that some physicians are atheists. It is also true that some rabbis are atheists as well. But it would be a mistake to infer from this that either medical science or Judaism is atheistic. Indeed, the majority of doctors I know are religious, many deeply religious. So it is not true that all physicians are atheists. But could it be that medical science is atheistic nonetheless? It is possible; but from what DesAutels says about this, I remain unconvinced. She seems to set up a false dilemma when she says that (1) Christian Scientists are idealists who believe in God and (2) because physicians are not idealists they cannot believe in God. Does she mean to say that only idealists can believe in God?

If materialists believe that material substance is all that exists, and if God is an immaterial substance, then materialists will be atheists. And if the only two metaphysical views that can be held are idealism and materialism, then if physicians are not idealists—if they believe in the existence of matter that they can manipulate through medical techniques—then they must be atheistic materialists. But, as DesAutels acknowledges, a person can also be a dualist, that is, can believe that there is both a realm of matter and an immaterial realm. Physicians who regularly attend church services seem to be examples of people who are dualists, believing in the reality of both material and immaterial things.

There are, though, several kinds of dualism. One kind holds that there is an unbridgeable gulf between the realms of body and mind, between the realms of matter and spirit. On such a view, medicine would still be atheistic, at least according to DesAutels, even though individuals who happen to be physicians could be theists. According to this first kind of dualism, physicians would be experts about the material world, and they would leave to religious leaders the realm of the immaterial. Thus medicine could still be materialist even though physicians were dualists. But another kind of dualist, one not recognized by DesAutels, is a dualist who thinks that there can be interaction between the material and immaterial realms.

Whenever my paternal grandmother went to see a doctor, she used to pray that God would work through her physician to heal her. Although she had a strong belief in the power of prayer, she thought that there needed to be an intermediary between the spiritual world and the realm of her sick body. Such an intermediary was provided when God worked through her physician to cure her sick body. This view may be ultimately indefensible philosophically. But this is not the issue. The issue is whether medical science must be understood to assert that because it is expert in healing the body it must be atheistic. I see no reason to dismiss the possibility that medical science is dualistic in the way that my grandmother was. I know many physicians who think that they effectively work "miracles" when they bring dying patients back from the brink of death. Indeed, it is apparently not uncommon for physicians to pray for the speedy recovery of their own patients, that is, that God will work "miraculously" through the doctor's own hands. Because one can either take this interactive dualistic view or not, medical science is simply agnostic about religious views, and hence there is no intractable metaphysical issue at the center of the dispute between Christian Scientists and medical scientists.

Medical science is not materialist, secular humanist, or atheistic. For this reason, the gap between Christian Scientists and medical scientists is not as wide as DesAutels would have us believe. And for this reason, the dispute between these two groups is not as intractable as DesAutels claims. Most physicians in my experience understand, and even believe in, the power of prayer. Physicians are not dismayed at Christian Scientists because they cannot understand people who believe that prayer can cure them. Rather, physicians are generally dismayed at Christian Scientists because they seem to be convinced not only that medical science has no power to cure the sick but that appealing to medical science can only make things worse for those who are suffering. Such a failure of understanding may have metaphysical roots, but it is not as intractable as failures to understand one another because the disputants hold opposite metaphysical views about the role of God in the world.

Socialization and Coercion

My proposal calls for respect and tolerance of the views of both parties to this dispute. Specifically, I propose that medical practitioners should not try to pressure Christian Scientists to accept their authority except in the most extreme cases and that Christian Scientists should be more open to medical diagnosis and treatment in those cases in which Christian Science appears not to be working for their deathly ill children. DesAutels is critical of my suggestion that the best way to accomplish this goal is to socialize each community to be more sensitive to the other. She contends that my call for what should be done, especially changes in socialization directed at the Christian Science community, amounts to coercion. In this section of the chapter I sketch a response to this charge.

Several times DesAutels embraces one of the main conclusions I advance in chapter 5. She says, "It is in accordance with Christian Science teaching and an expectation within the Christian Science community that a child be taken to a physician when a child's condition is not being adequately addressed using Christian Science." She also says that Christian Scientists should "take special care to notice when and if a Christian Science approach is not working in the case of children." In this we agree. So where is the disagreement? Only in DesAutels's estimation that no changes in current socialization of Christian Scientists or medical scientists should be made. But then the question is this: How will Christian Science parents know whether they should take their children to a medical specialist, and what will ensure that the medical practitioners they see will not instantly appeal for a court order to gain temporary custody of the child so that they can do whatever they want according to the medical conception of what is good for the child?

My proposal about socialization was not meant to countenance coercion. It was meant to be a call for a constructive change in the way both of the parties to this dispute educate their members to regard the other. The problem is that an impasse now exists: Christian Science parents are very reluctant ever to consult with a physician for fear that the physician will simply try to take over the care of their children. And medical practitioners are very reluctant to trust Christian Science parents to do what is best for their children because they do not understand the motives of the Christian Science parents in not seeking the full support of modern medicine. If fledgling members of both groups could be educated more fully about the beliefs and motives of the other group, then perhaps greater trust would arise between these groups and certain tragedies could be avoided.

DesAutels can find no good reasons for a Christian Scientist to agree to such a change in education or socialization because she sees the dispute as rooted in an intractable metaphysical dispute. As a result she cannot conceive that I can be proposing anything more than coercing Christian Scientists to change their metaphysical view and become believers in materialist, atheistic medical science. I have tried to indicate here that this is not my view. Surely, not all forms of education are coercive; or if they are, then the coercion is, at least in some cases, a benign coercion. Proposals to change grammar school curricula to include multicultural issues are often claimed to be an attempt to coerce people to be more tolerant of one another. It is indeed difficult to teach tolerance. But the hope is that education and socialization efforts aimed at multicultural issues can lead people to come to see the value of tolerance and to change their views of one another on their own. It is in this spirit that I proposed changes in socialization as a way to resolve the dispute between Christian Scientists and medical scientists.

The Problem with Children

There is quite a difference between what adults decide to do to themselves and what adults decide to do to the children who are under their care. We might be appalled by a religion that countenanced suicide rituals for its adult members while considering these adults' behavior vis-à-vis their religion none of our business. But things change radically when children are involved chiefly because children are generally not yet able to give voluntary, informed consent to what their religion demands of them.[2] When a religion seems to act in a way that is contrary to the best interests of its children, intervention is at least justifiably contemplated on the ground that each of us has a duty to rescue nonadults whose lives are imperiled.

The burden of proof is on the religion to show why such intervention should not be made when that religion seemingly imperils the lives of its children. Because of this, we should not give overriding weight to Christian Science parents in this dispute. Since Christian Scientists cannot prove that medical science will not cure their sick children, they should not be allowed to override such care, especially in extreme cases when nothing else seems to be working. Since medical scientists cannot prove (nor would most want to prove) that prayer cannot cure, they should not be allowed to override attempts by Christian Science parents to cure their children through these means. Overriding weight should only be given to the children's interests. What we need is a compromise in which all options are left open for the sake of the children.

The difficulty is that some Christian Science parents sincerely believe that if they even consult physicians they will do harm to the health of their children. So in good conscience they stay away from all doctors, no matter how sick their children are, and even when their Christian Science practices seem to be failing. This results in what is surely a tragedy: Children die who might have been saved. DesAutels is correct to point out that I am partially biased in this dispute in that I believe that medicine does have curative powers. At this point, a variation of Pascal's wager enters into the dispute. It seems foolish not to try medicine when all else seems to be failing, just as Pascal thought it foolish not to believe in God if one was not sure whether there was an afterlife or not.[3] In order for Christian Scientists to feel free to pursue medical means when all else seems to fail, they need to have more trust in physicians than they have now, and for this to happen physicians need to act in ways that merit this trust. My compromise is that we try to inspire both sides to trust each other, not blindly, but at least so that they can cooperate in those last resort cases in which, perhaps, medical science can prevent the death of a child. For the sake of the children it is at least worth a try.[4]

Notes

1. I am not claiming that the Christian Science religion endorses anything like this. It is interesting, though, that some medical practitioners I know believe that this is effectively what Christian Scientists condone when they refuse to allow their children to be subjected to lifesaving medical treatment.

2. For more on this topic, see the paper I coauthored with Hugh LaFollette, "Suffer the Little Children," in *World Hunger and Morality,* ed. William Aiken and Hugh LaFollette, 2d ed. (Upper Saddle River, N.J.: Prentice-Hall, 1996), 70–85.

3. I would also argue, again by appeal to a variation on Pascal's wager, that it would be foolish not to try to cure through prayer, regardless of one's religious views, if it became clear that medicine seemed to be failing to cure a sick child.

4. I am once again grateful to Peggy DesAutels for inspiring me to think hard about an issue that gets more complicated, and more philosophically interesting, the more I examine it.

8

Protecting Christian Science from Medical Science

Peggy DesAutels

In chapter 7, Larry May asks us to consider a minority religious group with practices and views much more unorthodox than those of Christian Scientists. Each year this religious group sacrifices one prepubescent member of the religious community on the altar of its main church on October 31. May's concern is that my arguments for giving Christian Scientists an unqualified right to practice their religion would, when applied more generally, lead to society's tolerating *any* minority group, no matter how morally reprehensible that group's values and practices. Nowhere, however, do I endorse the view that just any value system held by a minority group should be given overriding weight in our society. Instead I stress that minority groups holding views that challenge the underlying assumptions held by the majority are difficult for the majority to understand, give equal weight to, or fully respect. I argue that the only way two groups, in this case medical professionals and Christian Scientists, can determine whether and in what ways to compromise is first to consider *equally* the beliefs and value systems of both groups.

May and I would agree that an unorthodox minority group engaging in practices that appear to intentionally harm or kill its children should at least be challenged to explain how such apparently harmful practices are morally justified. (Surgeons appear to harm children when they cut into them, and some children even die while "under the knife"; but such cutting practices may well be morally justified.) If it is determined that a group is morally unjustified in engaging in practices that include intentional or systematic harms to children, such a group should be restrained from doing so. Whether or not there are morally justified reasons for intentionally harming or killing children makes for an interesting discussion, but it is not a discussion relevant to Christian Science refusal cases. Christian Scientists neither intend to harm nor intend to sacrifice their children. Thus May's comparison of Christian Scientists to a religious group that sacrifices children is misleading at best.

One of the main points made in this volume, at least as far as I am concerned, is that details do matter. The more one examines the beliefs and practices of Christian Scientists, the more complex their "refusals of medical treatment" become. Throughout this book, I make a series of detailed arguments that draw on the particulars—both value and belief particulars—attributable to the worldviews held by Christian Scientists and by those who are more medically minded. I note that *both* Christian Scientists and medically oriented individuals value health and well-being in themselves and their children. I note that members of *neither* group are ethically required to avail themselves of medical professionals or to continue medical treatments that prevent them from achieving their particular health-related aims. I explicate how these two groups differ over metaphysical assumptions, and then I explain why certain medical treatments and the assumptions underlying them are in conflict with Christian Science approaches and assumptions. Only after carefully considering the specific assumptions and practices of both Christian Scientists and physicians do I argue that medical professionals should accommodate a Christian Scientist's health care wishes.

Throughout my chapters in this volume, I have emphasized that medical science and the practice of medicine rest on secular materialist assumptions, whereas Christian Science and the practice of Christian Science rest on religious idealist assumptions. Larry May finds this assertion problematic. According to May, I seem to set up a false dilemma when I say that Christian Scientists are idealists who believe in God and that physicians are not idealists and thus cannot believe in God. I acknowledge that many individual physicians believe in God, that some physicians recommend prayer as a supplement to medical treatments, and that some physicians believe that God works through them. But the *practice of medicine* and the assumptions underlying this practice do not yet contain God-based treatments or explanations. More importantly, in clinical contexts, physicians put their primary faith in medicine and do not advocate (nor should they) approaches that *conflict* with medical ones, be they spiritual or otherwise. If a medical approach has even the slightest chance of working, no physician qua physician would recommend a spiritual approach *over* a medical approach. If either a physician or a patient happens to hold the view that

God works through physicians, this view is not the view of medical science. My point is and continues to be that although both Christian Scientists and medical practitioners value health and well-being, the conflicting practices within Christian Science and medicine rest on conflicting metaphysical assumptions.

As Larry May correctly notes, physicians are not dismayed when patients pray to be cured while continuing medical treatment. Rather, they are dismayed when patients pray *in place of* continuing medical treatment. Physicians view and treat disease biologically. Christian Scientists do not. According to May, there is no "intractable metaphysical issue" at the center of the dispute between Christian Scientists and medical scientists. His claim rests on the premise that it is possible to believe both in God and in doctors. May's grandmother did. And because Christian Scientists believe in God they can, and therefore should, also accept the view that God can work through doctors. At least I assume that this is how May proposes to reach a metaphysical compromise. But the Christian Scientist view of God and God's relationship to His creation differs from the view held by May's grandmother. In the Christian Science view, God is spiritual and knows only spiritual ideas. God does not know the human particulars about anyone, including doctors, but sees and knows His spiritual ideas only as perfect and eternal. The underlying metaphysical conflicts that exist between those who place their faith in doctors and those who place their faith in Christian Science are indeed intractable.

Some of May's proposed *practical* compromises between medical professionals and Christian Scientists are quite appropriate and would be perfectly acceptable to most Christian Scientists. But others are neither appropriate nor acceptable. For instance, one of May's more acceptable suggestions is educating "fledgling members of both groups" more fully about the beliefs and motives of the other group. Christian Scientists would agree that both groups should promote mutual respect and understanding. They would especially agree that medical professionals should know more about the beliefs and motives of Christian Science patients. But as a minority group living in a very medically oriented society, Christian Scientists are already well aware of the beliefs and motives of medical professionals. In fact, Christian Scientists highly respect the motives of most medical professionals and strongly support non-Christian Scientists' availing themselves of medical treatments when they view such treatments as their best option.

I do not, in general, consider education about another group's belief and value system (i.e., a multicultural approach to education) to be tantamount to coercion. But May does not merely recommend that Christian Scientists and medical professionals increase their understanding of and respect for each other's differences. He proposes that Christian Scientists be "socialized" into obtaining more medical diagnoses and treatments and, under certain circumstances, "pressured" to accept medical authority. May distinguishes socialization from coercion by claiming that socialization is merely "meant to be a call for a constructive change in the ways both parties educate their members to regard the other." But notice that elsewhere May does not ask simply that Christian Scientists and medical professionals be better educated about each other's motives, aims, and practices. He also asks that Christian Scientists be socialized to *alter* their own values and their own health-related practices in ways that Christian Scientists themselves do not choose to have them altered.

May appears to think that there are morally compelling reasons for the medical majority to educate the Christian Science culture out of some of its own values and practices. Certainly, there are a number of morally acceptable and noncoercive ways for one group to attempt to convert another group to its way of thinking. But whenever a majority culture attempts to "educate" a minority culture out of its beliefs against that minority culture's wishes, such attempts can easily slip into coercive attempts. At the extreme, Christian Scientists could be compelled by the majority to attend certain classes, or the Christian Science Church could be legally compelled to offer certain "educational" programming. When "education" becomes to any degree coercive, May has the burden of proof to show that such "educational" practices are, indeed, morally justified.

"Pressuring" can also be coercive. If by "pressuring" a Christian Science patient, May simply means that a physician should offer additional explanations and further education, then I would agree that such "pressuring" is morally acceptable. But "pressuring" by definition means something stronger than mere explanations and involves the threat of some sort of compulsion, constraint, or disciplinary action. The threats (overt or implied) inherent in pressuring, and thus its coercive nature, are especially salient when the person (or institution) doing the pressuring is in a position of power. Notice that Larry May advocates pressuring Christian Science parents to switch to a medical approach under certain circumstances but does not recommend pressuring medically oriented parents to switch approaches when medicine is failing.

I agree fully with May that Christian Scientists as a group and medical professionals as a group should talk more with each other. If I felt otherwise, I would not have agreed to cowrite this volume. Such discussions are not coercive. But some ways of pressuring members of a minority group to switch to the majority's way of thinking, even when such pressuring ostensibly occurs only under "extreme" circumstances, are coercive, especially when the group doing the pressuring has an inordinate amount of political, economic, and epistemic power.

In many ways, Larry May and I are in agreement on how issues surrounding the children of Christian Scientists should be handled. I agree, for example, that Christian Scientists as a group should be especially responsive to society's general concern over the well-being of children. I agree with May that medical scientists "should not be allowed to override attempts by Christian Science parents to cure their children through [prayer]" and that "overriding weight should be given to the children's interests." I agree too that "in order for Christian Scientists to feel free to pursue medical means when all else seems to fail, they need to have more trust in physicians than they have now, and for this to happen physicians need to act in ways that merit this trust." And finally, I agree that "physicians should find ways to cooperate with Christian Science parents in last resort cases." For someone who is medically oriented, Larry May is exceptionally tolerant of and accommodating toward Christian Science parents and the nonmedical health-related choices they make for their children.

I would like, however, to discuss May's assertion that "there is quite a difference between what adults decide to do to themselves and what adults decide to do to the children who are under their care." This difference, according to May, is due primarily to the fact that "children are generally not yet able to give voluntary, informed consent to what their religion demands of them." First, I consider it important to differentiate between younger children and adolescents. It is becoming increasingly acknowledged within the bioethics literature that most adolescents between ages fourteen and seventeen are capable of making even the most difficult of health care decisions for themselves.[1] Certainly most children of Christian Scientists within this age-group are capable of deciding whether they wish to use a Christian Science approach.

But even young children in families whose identity and entire way of life are inextricably tied to their religions should not be treated any differently from the adults unless it can be shown that such children are intentionally and systematically harmed by their families. The Christian Science approach to healing is taught and integrated into a child's life from a very young age. For example, when a child scrapes a knee, a Christian Science parent teaches the child to "look away" from the "false" material evidence and to think instead about the "truth" that she or he is God's perfect idea surrounded by God's goodness and embraced in God's ever present love. The children of Christian Scientists are not the passive recipients of health care practices done "to" them. Rather, they are taught how to pray, expect healing as a result of this prayer, and actually experience the expected results. Even the young children of Christian Scientists are actively involved in prayerfully responding to inharmonious situations of all sorts. Because children are taught the Christian Science worldview and are active participants in the Christian Science way of life, the same metaphysical conflicts experienced by Christian Science adults in medical settings will be experienced by the children of Christian Scientists. And even though many young children are not yet capable of making abstract and cognitively complex decisions, most young children of Christian Scientists would prefer, when asked, to use the approach consistent with their upbringing, as opposed to a very foreign and conflicting approach.

I do not mean to say by this that the children of Christian Scientists are *always* better off avoiding medical settings. I merely mean to point out that the best interests of a young child being brought up as a Christian Scientist will usually coincide with the interests of adult Christian Scientists. The decision to switch to a medical approach, even in extreme situations, is not a decision that Christian Scientists ever make lightly. May's suggestion that Christian Scientists use a variation of Pascal's wager in children's cases does not work here, especially if the idea is that one might as well "bet on" both medical and Christian Science approaches in children's cases. For the sake of their children, Christian Scientists, in good conscience, teach their children to approach life and health just as adult Christian Scientists do.

Notes

1. For a concise summary of the ways in which adolescents are being given increasing roles in their own health care decision making, see Robert F. Weir and Charles Peters, "Affirming the Decisions Adolescents Make about Life and Death," *Hastings Center Report* 27, no. 6 (December 1997): 29–40.

Conclusion: Agreeing to Disagree?

Margaret P. Battin, Peggy DesAutels, Larry May

In this volume, three philosophers concerned with the ethical issues that various forms of organized religion can raise have explored dilemmas posed by the beliefs and practices of Christian Science. One of us, Peggy DesAutels, was raised in the Christian Science tradition; the other two of us, Peggy Battin and Larry May, are not members of this tradition and hence view it from the outside, as indeed most critics do. But this is not a battle between adherents and critics; on the contrary, all three of us are trying to reach a conscientious, responsible, joint understanding of the difficult issues Christian Science raises and to recommend workable, sensitive, broadly acceptable social policies.

But it doesn't seem to be working. There are deep differences here, differences that appear to remain even after our extended discussions. Battin still thinks that Christian Science ought to provide base-rate data and other kinds of confirmatory evidence for the healings it claims to have accomplished; only with such evidence, she insists, can people (Scientists and non-Scientists alike) make informed choices about how to protect their health. The same sort of information, Battin thinks, is necessary for making informed choices about the health care of children. DesAutels rejects these demands for empirical study, insisting both that such information is irrelevant to the practice of Christian Science and that attempts to gather such information would impose the medical model of health and disease on Christian Scientists. Meanwhile, May still thinks a compromise is possible in the matter of medical treatment for children, if both Christian Scientists and medical professionals are socialized to respect each other's convictions; this would in general permit parents to seek Christian Science healing for their children most of the time but mandate medical treatment for problems that are severe or life threatening. Again, DesAutels rejects

123

this. Furthermore, Battin and May do not identify the same issues in Christian Science as the centrally problematic ones, though both agree there are problems that are not resolved by DesAutels's answers, sensitive and understanding though they may be. It looks as though we three have hit bottom, so to speak, in plumbing the depths of our disagreement. The civilized thing to do, it may now seem, is to "agree to disagree": To recognize that these differences are irreconcilable and to find some more or less makeshift way of accommodating public policy and practice to this huge gulf.

But do we really disagree? After all, we hold many points in common—matters of basic philosophical, political, and public policy commitment. How we can disagree about anything substantial if we agree about all these things? The following list displays just some of the things we do agree about:

- that people's religious beliefs should be respected
- that prayer may be meaningful and important to those who engage in it
- that state intrusion into religion should be minimized
- that ill health (whatever that is) is undesirable
- that people have the right to make their own health care decisions
- that Christian Science is a long-established, cherished tradition
- that Christian Science parents care deeply about their children
- that children ought not be abused, injured, or caused to suffer or die
- that children ought not be allowed to die when they can be saved
- that legal battles over how Christian Scientist parents may treat their children are undesirable
- that the state acts appropriately in protecting vulnerable parties from abuse
- that some medical treatment is followed by "cure"
- that some Christian Science treatment is followed by "cure"
- that some medical treatment fails to produce "cure"
- that some Christian Science treatment fails to produce "cure"

If there is disagreement, DesAutels claims, it is at a deeper level, not just about facts and values at any superficial level but about basic issues in metaphysics. Christian Science sees a person as an expression of divine Mind, not matter, and the human body as shaped by the comprehension of each individual; non-Scientists see the human body as flesh and blood, a material substance animated by a nervous system and guided by intentions—an ordered, functioning organic system. For Christian Scientists, "disease" is misunderstanding; for non-Scientists, disease is physical disorder in an organic physical system. This is the conflict between religious idealism and secular materialism, twain that cannot meet.

But can we really disagree about the metaphysics of the human body? To be sure, the entire history of philosophy might seem to provide ample fuel for such disagreement: Plato, Berkeley, Kant, and Hegel are idealists or partly so, though in various ways; Epicurus and Lucretius, Hobbes, Marx, and Darwin are materialists, though of different sorts too, and they have radically different theoretical views about the human body. But does the practical disagreement that erupts for us in friction over foregoing conventional health care in favor of Christian Science healing, and especially over denying conventional health care to children, resemble that of the philosophers?

Certainly, the disagreement is at least in part the product of what each of us, as believers or nonbelievers, as patients, as parents, sees as "out there," in the world, or "in here," in us and of us. But do we really "see" and experience something different? Three philosophers are writing this book; two of them stretch out their hands and see skin, flesh, the structure of bone; the third does the same but attempts to see the idea of God that lies behind this apparent physical structure. Democritus would have claimed to see his outstretched hand as a collection of atoms; Plato would have seen his as an exemplar of an ideal Form; many others thinkers would claim to see theirs in a variety of ways, though G. E. Moore stretched out his own hand hoping to end what he viewed as nonsense: "Is this a hand I see before me?" he asked, insisting that the answer could not be anything but yes.

It is right here that the most basic challenges and disagreements may seem to arise. Is the difference in what the three of us see as we discuss Christian Science, stretching out our hands before us, an elective difference, if it is a difference at all? Do "idealist" and "materialist" accounts provide accurate descriptions of what we each see and experience? Can one "choose" to see one's own hand in these different ways? Could one change one's way of seeing? (If not, presumably it would be impossible to "convert" to Christian Science.) Is "practical idealism" really possible at all? Or do we all actually see our hands as physical structures of skin, flesh, bone, with some of us—those with certain religious commitments—then "reinterpreting" this phenomenon as a manifestation of divine Mind, just as some philosophers reinterpret it as assemblages of atoms or instantiations of the Forms? Or perhaps is it the other way around; could we all be seeing our hands as projections of consciousness but reified by some of us as objects of flesh and bone? Of course there can be disagreements among people over all sorts of matters, including facts, policies, customs, beliefs, the requirements of morality, and many other things; but can there be genuine disagreements in practice, in everyday life, over metaphysics? Do we actually see and experience our own hands, our own bodies, in different ways, or do we merely live with different official commitments about how we will interpret them? Yet it is these very bodies, of which our hands are part, that are at issue in decision making about conventional medical treatment versus Christian Science healing.

If there are basic metaphysical disagreements, agreement may elude us. If there are not, we cannot "agree to disagree"; agreement itself is too near to let it drop. What might the agreement be, in practice, if we could reach it? Larry May suggests a compromise solution in which parents are free to employ Christian Science healing for their children's minor ailments but are expected to turn to conventional medicine for severe, life-threatening ailments, like Robyn Twitchell's intestinal blockage. Battin would accept this arrangement, provided that adequate base-rate and other data were available to show that conventional medicine outperformed Christian Science in severe, life-threatening ailments but not in minor ones, largely self-limiting ones, both for adults and children. Given such data, adults would be free as a matter of basic religious liberty to make whatever practical choices they wanted for themselves, even if it clearly meant a probable earlier death, but ought not make choices for their children that would likely mean death when recovery was otherwise possible. Could the Christian Scientist, DesAutels, agree? This might seem easy, since Christian Science can still flourish in the vast majority of cases in which the condition is not severe, iatrogenesis is a risk, outcomes are not known, or the condition is self-limiting; conventional medicine could be encouraged just in that minority of cases reliably known to be truly serious. But the Christian Scientist committed to an idealist conception of reality cannot agree without giving away the store; to agree to calling in conventional medicine for the most severe cases would be either to relinquish the claim that persons are "really" spiritual, idealist beings, not material ones, or to acknowledge that sometimes healing doesn't occur even in the best of attempts to see persons, including oneself, as ideal, spiritual beings. Of course, Christian Science already acknowledges that people are sometimes unable to fully understand the true nature of reality, and that hence prayer fails to achieve healing in some cases; but if it grants this, then the wisdom of "praying for a cure" is open to challenge in every case.

To see the issue more clearly of whether we can "agree to disagree," we can also explore whether we can or cannot agree in a specific case, for example, the case of little Robyn Twitchell. Clearly, we agree about a great deal. We all agree that Robyn's parents desperately wanted what was best for him. We all agree that Robyn's symptoms were, to the nonprofessional (though perhaps not to the professional), difficult to interpret: symptoms of serious distress intermittent with symptoms of apparent cure, confounded by the fact that his older brother had had similar symptoms the previous week and had recovered without incident. We all agree that Robyn experienced at least some pain, that he vomited, and that he died. Yet we disagree about what Robyn's parents should have done in responding to this situation. Battin thinks that the Twitchells should have been informed, when they first sought Christian Science healing, of the approximate likelihood that this treatment would be effective, given the symptoms, compared to conventional treatment, just as they would or should have been informed of the likely benefits and risks of conventional treatment: They should have been told that with surgery for the blockage there was a good chance that Robyn could have been saved and that without the surgery—with or without Christian Science prayer—he would almost certainly die. May thinks that the parents and the Christian Science practitioner who was called should have been socialized to recognize that the case was a serious one, appropriate for conventional medicine, and that Robyn should have been taken to the hospital. DesAutels thinks Robyn's parents did the loving, religiously sincere, appropriate thing for their child. Are we disagreeing about the facts of the case here, or are we really disagreeing about its metaphysics? Are we all just talking about differing interpretations of the evidence about what was wrong with Robyn, or are we talking about different conceptions of what Robyn's symptoms represented and indeed, about what Robyn, as a human person and human body, was in himself? If it is the former—different interpretations of evidence—we can agree to agree and keep working until we have all the facts and values sorted out; if is the latter—different underlying metaphysics—we can only disagree and perhaps not even agree on whether to do so or not. It may not even be easy to say what differences these alleged metaphysical differences would make, if any at all. There is no easy way to resolve these issues; it is what makes them so interesting, and it is why ethical issues in the practice of organized religion are so compelling, an area of philosophical reflection we all believe will grow.

Personal Note from Peggy Battin

In March 1998, distinguished clarinetist Christie Lundquist died. This is not a fictional story and this is not a made-up name; Christie Lundquist, first clarinetist of the Utah Symphony, was a clarinetist of national reputation, "legendary" in the words of one of her colleagues. I spoke with Christie only twice about her practice of Christian Science, but I had been watching for years from my balcony seat at the symphony. Over the years, she had grown thinner and a little gaunt, and the color of her skin had shifted from normal Caucasian flesh tones to a yellower, greener cast. Her colleagues in the symphony said that she missed many rehearsals, that she was often ill. We surmised that it was liver disease, ineluctably advancing.

A medically trained friend was with me at the symphony one evening and found her symptoms so pronounced that they could be diagnosed from the balcony. "She won't live six months," said the friend, but in fact Christie lived another three years; she was fifty-one when she died. Whether she would have lived longer (or not) with conventional treatment I do not know. A friend said that she had contracted hepatitis in Mexico twenty years earlier and that the national symphony with which she was playing had made her see a doctor; but of course she did not see a doctor and would not consider it. Her colleagues in the symphony were furious; she was a brilliant player as well as a remarkable athlete and a wonderfully witty human being. They loved her and they respected her, even though she seemed to have no conception of her disease or its potential consequences. Indeed, they said, among the woodwinds, she was always grabbing people's mouthpieces and trying them out.

Watching the progression of her disease from the balcony, performance after performance over a long period of years, cost an immense effort of will to try to summon respect—genuine respect, not superficial tolerance—for her beliefs and for her way of living. I too was angry: angry that her beliefs should lead her to die, destroying a remarkable talent, robbing the symphony of a brilliant player, and robbing herself of life. More than once, I wanted to rush down to the stage from the balcony and shake her, to say, "Christie, quick, go to a doctor before it's too late. Don't just let yourself die."

But when I talked with her, just once, and once again—seeing at close range the real deterioration of her skin, its many small lesions, the yellowed filaments in her eyes—she spoke so movingly of the importance of her beliefs that I could not bring myself to say words like "liver failure" or "see a doctor," which seemed not only rude and invasive but somehow irrelevant. She lived in a different world, I think, one in which these expressions would have made little sense. She told me at length how much her beliefs in Christian Science had contributed to her playing of the clarinet, and she seemed not at all afraid of whatever future she was facing. When she talked, I felt an odd sense of awe.

Those who spoke to Christie in the Christian Science nursing home in which she spent her final days said she was upbeat, very upbeat. She cheered them up when they called, they said, not the other way around, even though she knew she was dying.

Did Christie and I ever talk, really talk? Could she have conveyed to me at any real level what she believed or why she believed it? After all, I couldn't seem to talk to her about my own comparatively "materialist" conception of the universe or of the human body and its functions, and I couldn't seem to say the things I believed about her. I wanted to say, I can see that you are very ill; you should seek real medical help soon, before it is too late; it is stupid to waste your life this way. But I just couldn't do it. I do not know whether we could have ever really talked in any way that we both could have understood, in any way that would have resolved disagreement; but I know that it is too late now. I'm left with the anger—and the sense of awe. If there is a paradox and a deep gulf of understanding in approaches between those who believe in Christian Science and those who do not, this is it—that feeling of both intimacy and unbridgeable distance in this conversation between a nonbeliever who would go on living and a believer about to die.

Personal Note from Larry May

A doctor I know, perhaps the most open-minded and sensitive doctor I have ever known, was one of only two physicians on our hospital ethics committee to side with me in thinking that Christian Science children should not be forced into medical treatment. He and I often talked about how important it was to avoid paternalism in these matters. But one day things changed for him. Here is the story he told at one of our monthly ethics committee meetings. He had come to know a Christian Science child with cystic fibrosis who was referred to him by a doctor who had treated her since infancy. He eventually developed a "working relationship" with the family, agreeing never to discuss the child's medical condition with her and to do minor examination of her in her home every week. At least as he told the story, and I have no reason to disbelieve him, there was mutual respect between himself and the parents. When the girl improved he didn't see her for a few months, by mutual consent.

One day, the parents summoned him because the girl was not gaining weight and was breathing hard. At her bedside he detected a distinct blueness to her skin—she desperately needed more oxygen. He informed the family that she was seriously ill, slowly suffocating to death. He said he couldn't help her anymore in the restricted way they had been proceeding. He recommended immediate hospitalization. The parents refused.

He contacted our ethics committee and the hospital lawyer. He told us that he was beginning the process necessary to get a court order to force her parents to bring her into the hospital. He was clearly emotionally drained by the last few days, having had little sleep and worrying constantly. In our meeting, I argued with him (I was the only one), but my heart wasn't in it. For whatever reason, the doctor didn't pursue the court order, and the girl died several days later. Even though he did what I thought, at the time, was best, I'm still haunted by this story, as is he. The tragedy of the situation overwhelms me.

Personal Note from Peggy DesAutels

I could respond to the previous personal notes by describing cases either of Christian Scientists recovering from medically incurable conditions or of non-Christian Scientists suffering and dying while under medical care. I will do neither. I will simply add that I rejoice when others experience good in their lives and that I too am saddened when others suffer and die. Unfortunately, neither medicine nor Christian Science has found a way to eliminate suffering and death from human experience. All that any of us can do is attempt to find insight, health, and healing by turning to the sources we most trust.

Index

AAP. *See* American Academy of Pediatrics

Accommodation, 92, 100–101, 124

Addictive substances/behaviors: avoiding, 68; medicalization of, 99

Allard, Laurie: case of, 95–97

Allard, Shirley Andrew: prayer/study by, 96

Alternative healing systems: choosing, 38, 39; Christian Science as, 27, 29–30, 36n30, 46, 49, 53, 57; success rates of, 38, 40

American Academy of Pediatrics (AAP): child neglect and, 78; on Twitchell/Newmark cases, 82

American Nurses Association, code by, 92, 109

Anecdotal accounts, 37–38, 39, 40, 44, 57, 60, 64, 85; criticism of, 14–15, 38, 68; on failures, 16; qualitative information from, 63; sharing, 24, 45, 49

Assemblies of God, faith healing/conventional medicine and, 20

Attorneys, fiduciary obligations of, 26

Authority, 21, 83, 113; autonomy and, 80; challenging, 77–79; moral/practical, 91; parental, 80; in pluralistic world, 79–82; religious freedom and, 83

Autonomy, 31; authority and, 80; fiduciary principle and, 28; respecting, 25; restrictions on, 80; violation of, 10–11, 23–24

Base-rate information, 37, 39, 43–44; decision making and, 40; for non-self-limiting conditions, 17; providing, 35n20, 38, 123

Belief systems, conflict over, 93–95

Beneficence, 31, 78; fiduciary principle and, 28

Benjamin, Martin: on worldviews/beliefs, 93

Bible, Christian Science and, 5

Blood transfusions, refusing, 7, 12, 22, 26–27, 31

Blue Cross/Blue Shield, 46, 56, 60; Christian Science healing and, 27, 30, 39, 54, 62n2; reimbursement by, 12, 57

Burkitt, Sally: death of, 13

Calkins, Nancy, 72, 103

Canterbury versus Spence, 65, 66

Century of Christian Science Healing, A, 55

CHILD. *See* Children's Health-care Is a Legal Duty

Child neglect/abuse, 72; medical refusals and, 1

Children: health-related choices for, 3, 101, 114–15; medical treatment for, 16, 71, 91, 111, 120, 121–22, 124, 129; overriding weight to, 80, 115, 121; prayer/healing and, 122; rights of, 80, 81, 83

Children's Health-care Is a Legal Duty (CHILD), 36n24

131

About the Authors

Margaret P. Battin is professor of philosophy and adjunct professor of internal medicine, Division of Medical Ethics, at the University of Utah. She is the author, editor, or coeditor of thirteen books, including *Ethics in the Sanctuary* (Yale University Press), *The Least Worst Death: Essays in Bioethics on the End of Life* (Oxford University Press), *The Death Debate: Ethical Issues in Suicide* (Prentice-Hall), and *Physician-Assisted Suicide: Expanding the Debate* (Routledge), as well as a book in progress on global population growth.

Peggy DesAutels is assistant professor of philosophy, assistant director of the Ethics Center, and director of the medical ethics program at the University of South Florida. She conducts research and publishes in both biomedical ethics and ethical theory. She has published articles that have appeared in *Mind and Morals* (MIT Press), *Mother Time: Women, Aging, and Ethics* (Rowman and Littlefield), *Journal of Social Philosophy, Midwest Studies in Philosophy,* and *Philosophical Psychology.*

Larry May is professor of philosophy at Washington University in St. Louis. He has authored and edited a dozen books, including *Sharing Responsibility* (University of Chicago Press, 1992), *The Socially Responsive Self* (University of Chicago Press, 1996), and *Masculinity and Morality* (Cornell University Press, 1998). He teaches and writes in the areas of ethics, philosophy of law, and moral psychology. He has recently returned to school to get a law degree.